- ▶ What is the cure for all this FAT?

- ▶ The muscle chemistry of fat people is far different from that of fit people.

- ▶ It's a sad fact: the fat get fatter while the fit get fitter. BUT you CAN become one who burns fat efficiently.

- ▶ If you're not FIT, you're FAT.

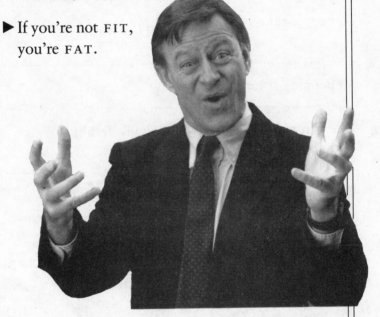

COVERT BAILEY shows you *how to change!*

ARE YOU

FIT?   OR

Fit people sink.

Fit people are fat-burners.

When fit people eat sugar, they make glycogen.

Fit people have lots of fat-burning enzymes.

Fit people eat more than fat people.

Fit people *use* fat efficiently.

When fit people exercise, it is usually aerobic exercise.

Fit people "waste" energy in everyday activities.

Fit people have long, lean, shapely muscles.

Fit people can be overweight without being overfat.

Exercise decreases hunger in fit people.

FAT?   SEE CHAPTER

T·H·E N·E·W
FIT OR FAT

Covert Bailey

Houghton Mifflin Company / Boston
1991

For information about permission to reproduce selections from
this book, write to Permissions, Houghton Mifflin Company,
2 Park Street, Boston, Massachusetts 02108.

Library of Congress Cataloging-in-Publication Data
Bailey, Covert.
    The new fit or fat / Covert Bailey.
      p.   cm.
    Rev. ed. of: Fit or fat? 1978.
    ISBN 0-395-60533-4
    ISBN 0-395-58564-3 (pbk.)
    1. Reducing exercises.   2. Aerobic exercises.   3. Exercise —
Physiological aspects.   4. Body composition.   I. Bailey, Covert.
Fit or fat?   II. Title.
RA781.6.B34   1991   91-10083
613.7'1 — dc20   CIP

Printed in the United States of America

BTA 10 9 8 7 6 5 4 3 2 1

Fit or Fat® is a registered trademark of Covert Bailey.

Contents

Foreword

WHEN EINSTEIN was asked whether he carried a notebook to put down his new ideas, he replied that he didn't get many new ideas. It appears that no one does. There is, as they say, nothing new under the sun. So when you are faced with a problem, it is best not to wait for inspiration. Chances are the solution lies not in a new idea but in a new look at an old one.

Covert Bailey, the author of *The New Fit or Fat*, has done just that with the problem of obesity. And he has found a solution by taking a new look at an old idea — exercise. "The ultimate cure for obesity," he states, "is exercise." Obesity departs as we increase our muscle mass and increase the muscle enzymes that burn up the fat and carbohydrates we eat. The way to do this — the only way we can do it, as Bailey points out — is to exercise regularly.

Bailey's whole emphasis is on fitness. He is not concerned with weight. He goes back to the dictionary definition of obesity as too much fat. People are not over*weight,* they are over*fat.* It is not weight that is crucial but the percentage of body fat. The higher that figure, the less lean body mass there is. The more fat, the less muscle. You can weigh 250 pounds and be virtually all muscle and bone or weigh 100 pounds and be overfat.

In recent years people have tried to control weight without looking at the percentage of body fat. The significance of that percentage in the development of obesity and the rationale of its treatment has been ignored. We have, however, begun to observe that most fat people actually eat less than skinny people. The endurance athlete, a lean, active creature, on the other hand, often eats insatiably yet gains no weight.

Our common sense, then, tells us that exercise keeps us slim. The idea that exercise melts off fat is part of our inherited wisdom. Still, scientists and nutritionists have never quite believed it. The whole idea goes against Newton's law of the conservation of energy. If it takes 10 miles of running to use up the 1,000 calories in a cheeseburger, milkshake, and french fries, exercise has to be an impractical method of losing weight. The scientific way to lose body fat must be to reduce energy intake, not increase energy putout.

Some researchers are having second thoughts about this traditional view. Dr. Eric Newsholmes of Oxford University has proposed that the exercised body develops what he calls "futile cycles." It acquires the ability to dissipate calories even in the absence of body movement, possibly through the production of heat. When an athlete rests, the wheels are still spinning, still using up energy in these futile cycles. Such cycling, says Newsholmes, may persist for two or three days after exercise or even more.

These cycles may contribute to other beneficial effects of exercise noted by Swedish investigator Per Bjorntrop. Exercise, he says, has a positive effect on obese people even when they are on unrestricted diets. Bjorntrop has documented decreases in hyperinsulemia, hypertension, and high blood fats. Obese people who exercise, he reports, undergo "a metabolic rehabilitation."

Apparently, exercise of the aerobic type causes a hypermetabolic state. When we jog or cycle or row or cross-country ski on a daily basis, all our functions are reset at a higher level. We now use the same amount of energy at rest that other people do when they are moving. We are no longer spectators gaining fat; we have become athletes losing fat.

Diets will not do this. Dieting loses muscle as well as fat. Dieting produces haggard people who do not look good or feel good either, as Bailey is quick to point out. He will have no truck with diets. Men of average size, he claims, should eat no less than 1,500 calories; women, no less than 1,200. When an exercise program becomes intense, of course, this intake has to be increased.

Nor is Bailey impressed by pounds lost. When a person tells him that he or she lost twelve pounds on a diet, he asks, "Twelve pounds of what?" Some of it is fat, of course, but some is water — which means nothing. And some of it is muscle, which means that the dieter has actually lost ground rather than gained it. In fact, the person will gain weight more readily when the diet is stopped.

What then should you monitor if you are overfat and embark on an exercise program? First, do not keep checking your weight. You may even gain two or three pounds in the beginning because of increasing muscle mass. Bailey advises people to throw out the bathroom scales. Stop shooting for an ideal weight, he says; shoot for health instead. Become aerobically fit, and fat (and weight) will take care of itself.

Taking your resting pulse, especially on awakening in the morning, is a good way to follow progressive improvement in fitness. The change in body fat can be checked by body measurements, particularly the waist, hips, and thighs. These are better indicators of your improving fitness than your weight. Actual fitness tests, like the Cooper twelve-minute test, will tell you that good things are happening to your muscles and your muscle enzymes. When your muscles are tuned up, says Bailey, you have more stamina, more energy, more drive, all because you are utilizing your food better and converting less of it to fat.

Research may provide better explanations of the beneficial effects of exercise on obesity, but they will not change Bailey's basic premise. The choice is for fitness or fatness, to exercise or not to exercise. The ultimate cure for obesity is exercise.

George Sheehan, M.D.

THE NEW
FIT OR FAT

1

A Word from Covert

BILL COSBY does a skit about a gambler who loses at the black-jack table, slaps himself on the side of his head, and says, "I don't believe it!" He loses again and again, each time saying, "I don't believe it!" Cosby's beleaguered victim looks more and more foolish each time he says it. It's a great routine, but it sadly par-allels the weight loss game that some people keep playing over and over. They go up against the house — metabolism — trying to get a big and fast weight loss against all odds.

I said it thirteen years ago, and I'll say it again. You can't win at the weight loss game by dieting. It's medically and physiologi-cally impossible to lose three pounds of fat from the body in a week, let alone the five pounds some plans advertise. Here it is, thirteen years later, and we still are in a diet frenzy. Our "heroes" on television and in magazines are still giving us their own per-sonal diet success stories. Why, with all the information available to them, would they think that a crash diet would work? They may be smart, educated, rich, and aggressive, but apparently they are gullible when the diet people come around.

The ultimate cure for obesity is exercise. I stated it loud and clear in the first *Fit or Fat?* and gave plenty of explanations. Diets are not the answer. They don't improve metabolism. They don't improve your chemistry. The only way to improve metabolism is to exercise. Today these statements are even better documented than they were then. So why do people persist in trying bizarre quick-weight-loss schemes?

One of the chapters in the original *Fit or Fat?* was "Diets Do Not Work." I've included it again, just as it was, with a new title: "Diets Still Do Not Work." If you're a first-time reader, memorize this chapter! If you've read it before, read it again! Here we are, nearing the twenty-first century, and people are still diet-crazy. And now some of the fast-weight-loss diets have the nerve to call themselves "medically supervised." That's great. We should also medically supervise people who jump off bridges — very important to have a doctor handy afterward. If someone told me I'd better have a doctor around when I went on a new diet, I'd say, "Gee, if it's that dangerous, I'm not going to do it under ANY circumstances." In the long run, exercise is the ultimate cure for obesity. That was my basic statement thirteen years ago, and it still holds.

I wish I could get fat people to say to themselves, "I'm going to find a creature who is skinny and ask him, 'How do you stay so skinny? What do you do?'" Fat people should ask a fox, a deer, or even the family dog how he stays so skinny. It's because of exercise, exercise, exercise. It's *not* because of diet.

In my first book I concentrated on the issue of fat because I knew that would motivate people to do something. But we now know that the benefits of exercise go way beyond the simple loss of fat. Blood profiles change, sleeping patterns improve, bone becomes more dense, even some psychological problems can be fixed with exercise. We can prove that people who are fit live longer and that THE FITTER YOU ARE, THE LONGER YOU LIVE. Did you know that this is true even for smokers? Smoking will shorten your life, but if you are a fit smoker, you'll live longer than unfit smokers. That almost seems like a joke, but it is not.

We have found the fountain of youth: it's exercise. Think about how you will be living the last twenty years of your life. Exercise today will have a tremendous effect on those years. The magic of the fountain of youth is that IT KEEPS YOU YOUNGER

EVEN AS YOU GET OLDER. Exercise keeps you physically and mentally young even as the years pile up.

Readers of *Fit or Fat?* may notice that the explanations in the beginning chapters of this new edition haven't changed very much. I had a message then, and I want to repeat it now. Let me give you a suggestion. Say you have a friend who is about to embark on a goofy rapid-weight-loss diet. I suggest that you copy the chapter "Diets *Still* Do Not Work" and give it to him. Giving a friend the whole book might be taken as an insult. The friend thanks you but puts it on the shelf. He — or she — never gets around to reading it. But if you give him just those few pages of "Diets *Still* Do Not Work," you might be able to turn that person around. You might be able to prevent him from doing something foolish. Please don't make thousands of copies because my publishers will go absolutely crazy, but make one or two. Together, you and I might be able to influence your friend.

Maybe you have a friend who is thin but who jiggles. Suppose you know that your friend is really unfit, that excess fat under the skin is causing the jiggling. You might give him Chapter 6, "Overweight versus Overfat." Don't say where it came from; just hand your friend those two pages. He might say, "Wow! I never thought of it that way. I may be skinny and fat, too!" This chapter would also apply to a friend who happens to be one of those big, heavy-duty people — someone who is very strong but who, everyone says, is fat. Maybe he isn't fat at all. Maybe he sinks to the bottom of the pool even though he weighs more than the doctor's charts say he should. You might stop him (or her) from needless, and useless, dieting with a couple of pages from my book.

Another possibility is Chapter 2, "Fat People Eat Less Than Skinny People." Perhaps you have a friend who beats herself up because she overeats, who says, "I just can't control my diet. I overeat and overeat." You know that person doesn't even eat as much as you do, yet she just doesn't realize it. Give her that chapter and see what comes of it. Sometimes if you start with a chapter, then follow up with the whole book, people will be ready to read it cover to cover.

Let me give you another suggestion. At the beginning of this book is a chart called Are You Fit or Fat? It contains facts about the differences between fit people and fat people. The two are very, very different. Give that to a friend who thinks being fit doesn't really do anybody any good. If you know someone who is still that ignorant, maybe this chart will trigger him to rethink his attitude and ask for more information.

The New Fit or Fat is exciting for me. I hope it will change people. I've already affected 2 or 3 million people, and I would like to get another 10 million if I can.

Don't accept the pessimism of newspaper articles that say only 10 percent of Americans are exercising. What such articles overlook is that only 5 percent of Americans USED to exercise. People are changing fast and furiously. Probably 90 percent of the public knows that they SHOULD exercise. If you ask people on the street if exercise is as good as it's cracked up to be, most will say yes. All of them know that it helps to control weight, and most people can list a dozen other benefits. Those who used to exercise will tell you that when they did, they felt better, slept better, and were less tense, and they wish they could get started again.

Don't tell me that we aren't having an effect. Americans are learning where the fountain of youth is.

2

Fat People Eat Less
Than Skinny People

MOST FAT PEOPLE feel guilty! Society points its finger in accusation at the overweight, making them feel that they are somehow morally weak, that they are gluttons with little strength of character. They chastise themselves at every meal, certain that they are overeating again. Nothing could be further from the truth. The will power of fat people never ceases to amaze me. They live a life of perpetual self-denial. If naturally skinny people denied themselves the way fat people do, they would fade away completely.

The truth is, most fat people eat less than skinny people.

During the initial interview in our clinic, fat women quickly tell us that they know why they are fat. They are convinced that they eat too much. When we ask the typical fat lady if she eats more than other people, she answers that she eats more than anyone. But when we ask her about her husband's eating habits, she explodes in exasperation, "That darn man eats three or four helpings at every meal and is still as skinny as a beanpole!" About this time she recognizes her inconsistency. Her husband eats far more than she does. She may then insist that she snacks during the day, which is probably the truth. Most nutritionists (who ought to know better) believe this is, in fact, the cause of her problem. But studies have confirmed that fat people are usually quite restrictive in their diets; they eat less than their skinny spouses. The simple truth is, the internal chemistry of fat people has adapted to low-calorie intake. And when they *do* overindulge, as all of us do from time to time, they gain weight while their skinny friends stay slim.

3

Diets *Still* Do Not Work

IT'S ALMOST IMPOSSIBLE to read anything these days without another diet staring you in the face. At the supermarket checkout are the inevitable ladies' magazines, each with a brand-new diet, guaranteed to make you slim forever. The book racks are filled with new books with bright covers pushing new diets, and they too guarantee that you can become a slenderella. There must be ten new, supposedly foolproof diets promoted every day. Usually the book makes the claim — in bold type where you will be sure to see it — that you can eat all you want of the foods you like. After all, who wants to read about a new diet that expects you to give up good foods when you are probably doing that already?

Well, you can take heart, because the diets that tell you to give up the foods you like don't work. They don't work because none of the diets work. It should be obvious that when ten new diets are published every day, each one claiming to be perfect, something fishy is going on. The problem is that diets don't work in the first place. THERE IS NO DIET NOW, AND THERE NEVER WILL BE A DIET, THAT CURES AN OVERWEIGHT PROBLEM. The reason for this is that diets don't attack the fundamental problem of the fat person.

You see, most people think that losing weight is the basic

problem. The fat person says, "I just can't lose weight." But when you ask the typical fat person if he has lost weight on any of the diets, he will tell you of the thirty pounds he lost on this diet and the twenty pounds he lost on that. In fact, many of the people I have interviewed have lost a thousand pounds on various diet programs over the years. Clearly, losing weight was not their problem at all. In fact, most fat people make a profession of losing weight. Not only do they lose weight very easily, they lose on practically every diet they try.

Sure, diets help people lose weight, but losing weight is not the basic problem. The problem is — gaining weight! Fat people gain weight easily and quickly, so they soon have more fat than they have just lost. Someone once said, "The American public has been dieting for twenty-five years — and has gained five pounds." Fat people who are constantly dieting should be asking themselves, "Why do I gain weight so easily?"

Suppose you had a broken leg and your doctor treated it simply with a shot of painkiller and sent you home. When the painkiller wore off, you would realize the doctor hadn't treated the basic problem. He should have set your leg in a cast. Well, that is what we do when we diet away our fat. When we finish a diet, we may have lost some fat, but our tendency to get fat is still there. The problem is that something inside is making us gain weight faster than other people do. Something in our body chemistry is favoring the deposit of fat.

When a naturally skinny person eats 1000 calories, all of them get burned, wasted, or somehow used up. When a fat person eats 1000 calories, perhaps only 900 of them are used up and the remaining 100 are converted to fat. For years, nutritionists have explained this with the observation that fat people exercise less. Well, that isn't the whole story. The fat person's body adjusts somehow to the making of excess fat.

In conclusion, yes, fat people may need to use a diet to help them lose excess fat. But dieting is only a superficial solution. The real cure is to find a treatment that changes their body chemistry so they won't have such a tendency to make fat out of the foods they eat. They need to find a way to avoid getting fat all over again. There *is* a way every person can alter his chemistry so that fewer calories are converted to fat. The superfat won't become superskinny, but everyone can improve a little.

4

The Body Machine

FOR YEARS there has been one standard answer for overweight people; you eat too much, or you exercise too little, or both. Doctors, nutritionists, and dietitians all echo the "party line." Well, it simply isn't true! There are people who get fat easily and people who remain skin and bones no matter how much they eat or how little they exercise. Not only can two people differ radically in their tendency to get fat, but the same person can change radically in his lifetime. Women who take birth control pills often gain more easily. The party line would be that they started to eat more or exercise less, but thousands of women claim the contrary.

The traditional approach to overweight can be shown by a drawing of a water tank. Water is added to the tank by a faucet above and let out of the tank by a faucet below. Humans are supposed to be just like this tank. Increasing the flow from the upper faucet is like eating more calories; when you do, the level in the tank goes up. Closing the lower faucet is like decreasing your daily exercise; the level of fat in your body goes up. Well, this analogy is partly true; getting fat is largely a matter of eating too much and exercising too little. Unfortunately, the analogy breaks down under practical everyday experience because it implies that people are passive reservoirs, affected only by outside food supply and exercise.

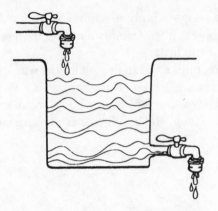

The fact is, we are not passive reservoirs or tanks, but active metabolizing machines, each different, each handling calories differently. I prefer to think of the body as a machine that runs efficiently or inefficiently, depending on circumstances. Just as an automobile may be tuned up properly to get more mileage from its fuel, the human machine also can become more efficient.

One of the unique features of the human machine is that it has two fuel tanks: one tank for sugar or, more technically, glucose and one for fat. Wouldn't it be neat if our cars were built the same way? Anytime we ran out of gasoline, we'd just switch over to our diesel fuel tank. Actually, in our bodies, we don't switch back and forth from one fuel to another; we use both simultaneously.

Most people are unaware that 60–70 percent of the energy muscles need when one is resting is supplied by fat. That is, fats, either from a recent meal or from fat deposits, travel through the blood to muscle, where they contribute more than half of the resting muscle's energy needs. Glucose and fats are burned side by side all day long, but fats supply most of the energy.

Storage of fat is therefore a natural body function. The trouble is, fat people's bodies are overly proficient at storing fat and are less than normally proficient at burning it.

Our analogy with the tank of water doesn't hold completely

because some people's body machines work harder to store fat than other people's. It isn't simply a matter of "you eat too much or you exercise too little."

Furthermore, unlike the analogy with the water tank, being fat tends to make you get even fatter. Fatness is a vicious cycle; the more fat you have, the more your body chemistry, or metabolism, changes to favor the buildup of even more fat.

5

Fat Floats! How to Test Your Own Body Fat

IF YOU THROW a pound of butter in a swimming pool, it will float just like a cork. When oil tankers collide at sea, they spill oil, a form of fat, which floats on top of the ocean. The fat in your body is no different. The more fat you've got, the better you will be able to float in a swimming pool. When I was a boy, I had a girlfriend who could float so well that she could read a book while lying calmly on top of the water. One day she asked why I never floated. Naturally I told her I could float if I wanted to, I just didn't want to. Well, the truth is, when she finally got me to try, I sank like a rock. It made me mad, and I vowed that someday I would be able to perform this marvelous feat just as well as she. Well, eventually that's just what happened . . . I got fat.

In contrast to fat, lean muscle and bone do not float. Scientists call that part of the body the lean body mass. It is quite practical to think of the body as having two distinct parts, the fat part that floats and the lean body mass that sinks.

There are many ways to estimate a person's body fat, but by far the most precise method is based on how well one floats. We use a large water tank in which the person can be completely immersed while sitting on a pipe frame chair hung from a scale.

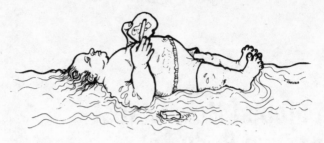

Fat floats!

The scale with its hanging chair looks much like the scale in the vegetable section of the supermarket. The more bone and muscle you have, the more easily you sink and the more you weigh under water. The more fat you have, the more you tend to float and the less you weigh under water. Big fat people approaching our water tank are afraid they will break our scale. But the truth is, the fatter they are, the lighter they are under water. Under water, it's the skinny people who weight the most. It sounds funny, but we compliment people who are very dense. To us, dense is beautiful.

The underwater immersion test is the most accurate method for determining body fat, and many universities use it in their physical fitness education programs. It involves some sophisticated equipment, so you can't easily do it in the backyard swimming pool. But there is a game you can try in a swimming pool, based on the same principle, that will give you an idea of your fat level. Have several people fill their lungs with air and float on their backs. Then, when someone signals "Go!" everyone blows his air out. Slowly, everyone should begin to sink. The one who hits bottom first is the leanest.

I once did this test with Carl, a very lean marathon runner. As I settled slowly on the bottom of the pool, I looked over at Carl. He had hit the bottom so hard that he had bounced up and was coming down a second time!

Above 25 percent fat, people float easily.

At 22–23 percent fat (healthy for a woman), one can usually float while breathing shallowly.

At 15 percent fat (low for a woman, healthy for a man), one will usually sink slowly even with a chest full of air.

At 13 percent fat, one will sink readily even with a chest full of air and even in salty ocean water.

These numbers are only approximate because one's floatability is also affected by age, lung volume, and water temperature. Underwater weighing isn't as simple as it sounds and can't be done accurately as a backyard operation.

There are several other techniques for determination of total body fat, most based on measuring the fat just beneath the skin, called subcutaneous fat. These methods assume that the amount of subcutaneous fat increases as total body fat increases; that is, as fat around the heart and lungs increases, fat under the skin will also increase. When you consider all the places inside the body where fat can accumulate (such as around the intestines and marbling inside muscles), it's hard to believe that measuring changes in skin fat would reflect changes in total body fat. The fact is, subcutaneous fat measurements provide amazingly accurate estimates of total body fat.

Skin fat can be measured by pinching it between the fingers, pinching it with a sophisticated caliper, bouncing ultrasound through it, or passing a special light through it. Accuracy of any of these methods depends on at least three important assumptions:

1. The number of places and the selection of places on the body.
2. The accuracy of fat determination in the skin at any one place. Obviously, pinching with your fingers is the least reliable.
3. In some people, the skin fat determination may NOT reflect their total body fat. In very fit people, total body fat is overestimated, and in very skinny but unfit people, it is often underestimated.

In our clinic we use skinfold calipers quite a bit because they are quick, cheap, easy to use, and surprisingly accurate. But I still prefer the water tank when it is feasible.

Authorities disagree somewhat, but I think it is safe to say that 15 percent fat for men and 22 percent fat for women are maximums for good health. Good athletes often have much lower percentages. Thin cross-country runners are often as low as 6 percent. When professional football teams have been measured, the heavyweight linemen have averaged about 17 percent and the faster-moving quarterbacks about 10 percent. The linemen, you notice, are slightly over our theoretical 15 percent because a little extra fat means extra weight and is presumably an advantage. But we question whether this is conducive to good health, since these are the men who "turn to fat" the quickest when they give up the sport.

The higher fat level in women, even those who are normal and healthy, may partially account for the greater incidence of obesity in women than men. Since women have more fat to start with, it's probably easier for them to get fatter.

These percentages, 15 percent for men and 22 percent for women, are the highest percentages one can have and still be considered in the normal range. We have measured thousands of people, however, and most men average 23 percent fat, most women 32 percent. Don't confuse *average* with *normal*. To be five or ten pounds overweight may be *average*, and all your friends may be the same, but that doesn't mean you're *normal*.

At this point, the question of body type often arises. You may reason that 15 percent and 22 percent are normal for mesomorphs, but shouldn't ectomorphs, the "naturally skinnys," be less than that? And shouldn't the endomorphs, the "naturally fatsos," be more? My answer is an emphatic no! All men should strive for 15 percent maximum fat. A 200-pound man can carry 30 pounds of fat, which is 15 percent of his weight. A 160-pound man should carry only 24 pounds of fat, which is also 15 percent of his weight. If a man has large bones and a lot of muscle, he can carry more fat without exceeding the 15 percent. His total weight can be greater than that of another man who is the same height and has slender bones, but they both should shoot for 15 percent fat or less.

I have seen many people who could have been called "naturally fatsos," but who subsequently brought their fat level down to a point where they didn't fit the endomorph label anymore. It is even more astonishing to find that many ectomorphs, who appear quite thin, even skinny, have a high percentage of fat.

Rather than use those terms to describe apparent differences in body type, I prefer to discard them completely in favor of fat percentages.

Body Fat Percentages
(underwater immersion testing)

	Men	Women
Fattest I've tested	55%	68%
Average American	23%	32%
Healthy normal*		
Oriental	18%	25%
Caucasian	15%	22%
black	12%	19%
Top athletes	3–12%	10–18%
Lowest I've tested	1%	6%

*There are racial differences in bone density. The bones of black people are heavier than those of Orientals, so they sink more easily in water. To allow for these differences, healthy Oriental men and women should be 18% and 25%, respectively, and healthy black men and women should be 12% and 19%, respectively.

6

Overweight versus Overfat: Some Overweight People Aren't Fat

MOST PEOPLE are concerned about being overweight, but the term is obsolete. We have said that overweight people are overweight because they have excess fat. But now we realize that fat can be hidden inside the body in such a way that you can be carrying a lot of excess fat without seeming overweight at all. Take, for example, the former weight lifter. Once he was very strong, with lean, hard muscles. Since giving up the heavy physical stuff, his muscles have fattened up somewhat. He may be the same weight as before, but now it's fat weight instead of muscle weight. He has become overfat without getting overweight.

The sad thing is that the same process has taken place in 90 percent of adult Americans. Up to the age of fifteen, the majority of us are very active, using calories as fast as we eat them. But then we "grow up." We settle down to the adult activities of drinking, working, and commuting in cars. Our muscles gradually become less dense, less lean, and more fatty.

A similar scene can be visualized with beef cattle raised on the range. Young calves romp and cavort, stopping only occasionally to nurse from their mothers. Gradually they settle down, and their wonderfully lean muscles "go to fat." With lack of hard use, the muscles develop those streaks of fat we call marbling. The more streaking (or marbling) of fat in the muscles, the more we prize the muscles as steaks.

Like beef cattle, humans become less active as they mature. Most of my adult clients mistakenly believe they are just as active, or perhaps even more active, as adults than they were as kids. But they are confusing different kinds of physical activity. I am talking about sports activities that really put muscles to work, that really stress muscles to capacity from time to time. Don't think of a long day of cleaning house, cooking meals, picking up after kids, or working on your feet at a job as real muscular activity. Such work may leave you exhausted at the end of the day, but to your muscles it is only busywork. Such routine daily work may never amount to more than 50 percent stress to your muscle; hence 50 percent of your muscle can atrophy, to be replaced by fat. Don't confuse work with exercise.

As fat seeps into your muscles, you may not gain weight because fat is merely replacing unused muscle. Most adults who weigh the same at forty as they did at twenty have nevertheless gotten very fat. We start to gain weight only when we have so excessively overeaten and underexercised that we exceed the capacity of the muscles to hold internal fat. Then the fat begins to deposit outside the muscles, under the skin. This fat is no longer replacing atrophied muscle but is adding to the body, and you get overweight. People who are just starting to get overweight are usually already overfat. If you are only five pounds *overweight,* you are probably at least thirteen pounds *overfat.*

To emphasize in another way the difference between being heavy and being fat, let me tell you a true story about a 285-pound football player. He was a valuable man on one of the big West Coast pro football teams, but each month his coach fined him for being overweight. He was only five feet ten inches tall, so his coach reasoned that he must be fat to weigh so much for that height. For a year or more, the big man dieted all the time, unsuccessfully trying to meet his coach's idea of ideal weight. Finally a university that was engaged in research on fat and physical performance agreed to determine the percentage of body fat of each player on the football team. To the amazement of all, our 285-pound man came out 2 percent fat, an astonishingly low number, considering that 15 percent fat for men is considered normal. Needless to say, his coach stopped fining him, and he stopped his starvation dieting. He gained weight to 325 pounds, which was a more normal fat content for him; he then felt much stronger and performed much better on the football field.

Here then is a case of confusing weight with fat. You can make no realistic determination of how fat you are by your weight.

My own life provides another example of the confusion between overweight and overfat. My case is the opposite of the football player's, and more typical of American fatsos. It also illustrates the worthlessness of the bathroom scales that we rely on so much. For the majority of my life, I have not fluctuated in weight. From the age of twenty to thirty-seven, I weighed 170 pounds, never varying more than a half pound. I was one of those obnoxious people who could eat anything and everything without the slightest change in weight. So when I started to gain weight rapidly at the age of thirty-seven, I was startled and looked hard for the cause of the change. Since my weight had been so steady for so long, it seemed obvious that I must have made some rather radical change in my life as I turned thirty-seven. Though I searched my own memory and questioned my friends, I could not discover any significant change at that time of my life. I considered possible emotional conflict, troubles at work, sickness, medications, smoking — everything. There was nothing I could put my finger on.

Then it occurred to me that perhaps a significant change had taken place a long time previously that hadn't hatched into a weight problem until I turned thirty-seven. And there was the answer! At thirty-two, I had had a most radical change in life style: I got a job. And with the job, I had money. I had huge business lunches, each with two or three drinks. At the same time, I gave up the extremely active sports life that had been my way before. You have to picture this — a trim thirty-two-year-old man drastically increasing his daily calories, including rich foods and alcohol, and at the same time equally drastically reducing his calorie expenditure. He would have to get fat, right? The party line says he would have to get fat. Well, *I didn't gain a pound for nearly five years.* So I thought I wasn't getting fat. In fact, I used to gloat in front of my business associates. Clearly, God intended that I would be eternally beautifully thin. And Then It Happened! I started gaining weight like everybody else.

From previous chapters it should be clear that I was really getting fat from the day of the big change when I turned thirty-two. But for nearly five years, the fat went into my muscles as the muscle itself atrophied from disuse. In other words, the fat replaced the muscle. With one thing merely replacing the other, I didn't gain any weight. I was getting fatter but not heavier. But muscles can hold only so much fat! In time muscular degeneration slows and calories deposit outside the muscle, under the skin. This subcutaneous fat is not replacing anything; it is simply an addition. So I gained weight. I got fat for five years before I started gaining weight.

7

What Is My Correct Weight?

IN CALCULATING your correct weight, we start with your lean body mass (LBM). We can't start with your age, your height, or your body type. The weight tables that your physician uses are based on several of these factors put together. Such tables were useful when nothing better was available, but it is clear now that they can be off by twenty to thirty pounds for any individual. It is possible to be overweight according to the charts and yet be underfat. And the reverse is true. We have measured many skinny people who are underweight according to the charts but overfat. They have no visible subcutaneous fat, but their muscles are loaded with fat.

We determine a person's ideal weight by the size of his frame, or lean body mass. If you have large bones and muscles, we would project a greater weight for you than for someone else of your same height who has thin bones and small muscles.

Male at 15% Fat*

Age	Total weight	Fat	LBM	Activity
20	170 lbs.	25 lbs.	145 lbs.	Wrestling
38	162 lbs.	24 lbs.	138 lbs.	Running
45	135 lbs.	20 lbs.	115 lbs.	Prison camp

*Male maintaining 15% body fat despite decreasing muscle mass as his activities change.

Let's take as an example a man at three different times in his life. When he is twenty years old, he is in college and involved in wrestling, gymnastics, and weight lifting. All three activities have added muscle to his frame, so his lean body mass is 145 pounds. He can carry 25 pounds of fat and weigh 170 pounds.

At the age of thirty-eight, he is a businessman whose only real physical activity beyond weekend skiing and some golf is running. The running keeps him lean and healthy, but it is not a sport that "packs on" much muscle. In fact, since upper body muscle is not needed for his sport, he will actually lose some of it. So now he has only 138 pounds of lean body mass. He shouldn't carry more than 24 pounds of fat and shouldn't exceed 162 pounds. His body adapts beautifully to its new role. Obviously, a runner doesn't need the upper body musculature of a gymnast. As muscle mass decreases, total weight should decrease also.

Let's take a third situation. Suppose our man, now in his forties, undergoes some extreme deprivation, such as two years of near starvation in a prison camp or perhaps a chronic debilitating disease for several years. He will lose much fat and much muscle. At the end of such hardship, he will be haggard and thin. His mother and probably his physician will want to fatten him up. I emphatically disagree. If his lean mass has dropped to 115 pounds, he should not carry more than 20 pounds of fat and shouldn't weigh more than 135. The only healthy recourse for such an individual is to replace the lost muscle, adding fat only to maintain 15 percent. If he eats to add weight, he will only add *fat* weight and will end up obese, just like the more typical fatso — even though he may still appear thin.

Most sedentary Americans show not only a decrease in lean mass as they grow older but also an increase in fat content.

Consider the changes in a sedentary woman. Let's say that at age twenty she is a healthy 22 percent fat and weighs 120 pounds. By age thirty-five she is proud that she has gained only 5 pounds, but she is, quite typically, 30 percent fat. If you look at the table on page 26, you will see that she has actually gained 12

Typical Body Composition Changes in a Sedentary Woman

Age	% Fat	Total weight	Fat	LBM	Ideal max. weight
20	22%	120 lbs.	26 lbs.	94 lbs.	120 lbs.
35	30%	125 lbs.	38 lbs.	87 lbs.	112 lbs.

pounds of fat while losing 7 pounds of muscle. Her lean body mass is now only 87 pounds, and to be 22 percent fat, she should not weigh more than 112.

You can see that the term "correct weight" is really quite ambiguous. A person's "correct weight" changes as his lean mass changes. If our sample woman exercises, she can rebuild her lean mass to the former 94 pounds and, in a sense, earn the right to weigh 120 pounds again. If she doesn't exercise, her correct weight is 112 pounds.

The amount of lean body mass you have also largely determines how much you should eat. After all, it's the lean body mass that burns up the calories. When you put gas in your car, it's the size of the engine that determines gas consumption, not the size of the car. For all practical purposes, the fat part of you doesn't need calories. You don't need to feed calories to your fat; fat *is* calories. Two people may weigh the same, yet one may have more fat, and therefore less lean body mass, than the other. If they both eat the same number of calories, the one with the smaller lean body mass will gain weight. In the next few years, calorie charts will become available telling you how many calories you can eat based on your pounds of lean body mass.

In calculating ideal maximum weight, we have to start with the part of you that functions, that all day burns calories, even when you are asleep. We have to start with the amount of active metabolizing tissue you have, your lean body mass. Then we calculate how many pounds of fat you can add to your lean body mass so that if you are a woman you would be 22 percent fat or, if you're a man, 15 percent fat. If you exercise in such a way that your lean body mass increases, your need for calories will increase, and you can carry more fat without exceeding the ideal 22 percent or 15 percent.

Pounds of Lean Body Mass (Frame Size) for Men

5'5"	5'6"	5'7"	5'8"	5'9"	5'10"
108–120	110–125	112–129	118–132	122–137	127–145

5'11"	6'0"	6'1"	6'2"	6'3"
133–153	137–163	140–168	143–176	145–183

Pounds of Lean Body Mass (Frame Size) for Women

5'0"	5'1"	5'2"	5'3"	5'4"	5'5"
70–86	73–89	75–91	78–93	81–96	83–99

5'6"	5'7"	5'8"	5'9"	5'10"
86–102	90–105	93–109	95–115	98–119

These charts represent the range of lean body mass of people I've tested who are in the healthy fat range of approximately 15% for men and approximately 22% for women. Unfortunately, I do not have enough data to give ranges for men shorter than 5'5" or women taller than 5'10" so these people must estimate their desirable lean body mass based on the height nearest their own. You can calculate your ideal total weight by dividing your lean body mass by .85 if you're a man and by .78 if you're a woman.

8

What Is the Cure
for All This Fat?

THE FIRST THING to do is to plant firmly in your head that the problem is not the excess fat, it's the lack of athletically trained muscle. Carrying an extra twenty pounds of fat isn't as bad as we have been told. Suppose you carried around a twenty-pound knapsack all day. Would that be bad? The extra load might be a strain on someone in poor physical condition, but if the weight were added slowly it might actually be a good way to get in shape. When I was on the ski patrol, skiing all day with ten pounds of first aid equipment didn't bother me at all. A few years later, when I was ten pounds *overweight,* I really noticed it. My point here is not that extra fat is good but that the lack of good muscle is bad. It's the underlying body changes accompanying the extra fat that do you in.

As muscle gives way to fat, not only does the actual quantity of muscle decrease, thereby decreasing the need for calories, but also the chemistry of the remaining muscle changes in such a way as to require fewer calories.

Dieting may decrease the weight of your knapsack of fat, but it cannot increase the amount of muscle or reverse the badly altered chemistry of the muscles. Dieting attacks subcutaneous fat first; it will remove intramuscular fat only under the most severe

prison camp circumstances. Even if you were willing to undergo such rigor, the results would be disappointing, because you
would have done nothing to prevent yourself from getting fat all
over again. Furthermore, you might have actually worsened your
situation; radical dieting, unbalanced dieting, shots, and fasting
have been shown to lessen muscle mass while you are losing fat.
In fact, there is good evidence now that one should get fit *before*
embarking on any kind of diet program. A well-exercised body
seems to respond more quickly and with less muscle loss to the
stress of dieting.

We have developed such a mania for losing weight that we
overlook what the lost weight consists of. Suppose I were to call
you on the telephone with the exciting news that the local supermarket was selling twelve pounds for only $1.29! Your reaction
would be, "Twelve pounds of what?" Well, that's my reaction
when someone tells me of a terrific diet that guarantees you
will lose twelve pounds in no time at all — twelve pounds of
what?

There are nationally known weight-watching organizations in
which a loss of weight is the only criterion of a member's success.
Unfortunately, while losing fat, the member may also be losing
muscle, which decreases the need for calories and augments the
problem. All of us can think of friends who have gone on diets
only to end up looking gaunt and haggard. We admonish them
and tell them they really would look better with a little fat on
them. But it isn't the loss of fat that gives them a wasted appearance, it's the muscle loss! Additionally, the loss of muscle and fat
through dieting does nothing to improve body shape. If the person was fat and pear-shaped before a radical diet, he'll end up
skinny and pear-shaped afterward.

Earlier I mentioned that many people who appear skinny are
sometimes high in fat. What most people do when they want to
gain weight is eat. And when one overeats to gain weight, the
added weight is only *fat* weight. The skinny person doesn't really
look more shapely with a gain in fat weight. The waistline dis-

appears, the shoulders narrow a little more, the thighs and buttocks fatten up, and a double chin may even develop. In other words, overeating to gain weight will only add fat and put it in places where you need it the least.

Compare these overeaters and undereaters to the many people who have exercised their bodies to low fat levels. They are full-bodied, healthy individuals who lead active lives without being constantly concerned about the number of calories they eat.

Exercise increases muscle, tones it, alters its chemistry, and increases its metabolic rate. All of these cause you to burn more calories even when asleep.

THE ULTIMATE CURE FOR OBESITY IS EXERCISE!

The most efficient exercise for this purpose is aerobic exercise. Briefly, aerobic exercise means steady exercise, exercise that demands an uninterrupted output from your muscles for a minimum of twelve minutes. It has been shown in many exercise physiology laboratories that steady, continuous exercise repeated every day reverses the syndrome of fat replacing muscle more quickly than any other kind of exercise. In other words, if you want to make muscle lean again while removing the marbled fat, you must replace the fat with lean muscle. This does not mean making big, bulky muscle such as the weight lifter wants. It does mean making lean again the muscle you already have. Most people don't want to do body building in the sense of weight lifting; they want the muscle they already have to be lean and functional. Steady muscular work for endurance does just that. As the muscle gets leaner, your metabolism changes automatically, and you burn more calories without even knowing it.

The word aerobic means air, specifically the oxygen in the air. The muscles need oxygen to function, and their need for oxygen goes up dramatically when we work them. We can measure how hard a muscle is working by how much oxygen it is using (or burning). As you exercise harder, you need more oxygen, and your heart rate goes up. The increase in your heart rate due to exercise is an indirect measure of how hard your muscles are working.

If you make a muscle work too hard, it will need more oxygen than your heart and blood can deliver. When muscles fail to get enough oxygen, they are working *anaerobically* (see Chapter 14). Aerobic exercises make the muscles work hard enough to need lots of oxygen but not so hard as to exceed the ability of the heart and blood to deliver it.

Exercise that is hard but not too hard and continuous for a minimum of twelve minutes, does more to increase fitness than other kinds of exercise. Aerobic exercise is the *most efficient* way to remove the marbling fat, which in turn is the most efficient way to change your metabolism so you won't get fat anymore. Anything we do that uses our muscles can be called exercise. And any exercise, even the household chores I made fun of earlier, helps to keep muscle intact. But to retain a full complement of muscle, we need exercise that uses it fully. Most people are limited in the time they can spend on an exercise program, and some would prefer not to exercise at all. So the shortest exercise of greatest efficiency should have wide appeal.

You can get as much benefit from fifteen minutes of jogging as from one hour of tennis. You can make your muscles perfectly lean by playing tennis, but you will have to play hard, two to three hours a day, six to seven days a week. For most people it would be much better to do a steady aerobic exercise every day for fat control and conditioning and then play tennis for fun!

The main criterion of aerobic exercise is that it be continuous and steady. We don't know exactly why that works, but it does. There is something about pushing a muscle to work hard at a steady pace that leads quickly to a firming of the muscle and a loss of its marbling. Stop-and-go exercises just don't do the same thing as quickly. There are very strong weight lifters who cannot run a mile and whose muscles are loaded with fat. These are people who "go to fat" if they become inactive.

The table on page 32 contains a list of steady endurance exer-

Aerobic and Nonaerobic Exercises

| | NONAEROBIC | | |
AEROBIC	*Stop and go*	*Short duration*	*Low intensity*
Running/jogging	Tennis	Weight lifting	Golf
Cross-country skiing	Downhill skiing	Sprinting	Canasta
Jumping rope	Football	Isometrics	
Running in place	Calisthenics	Square dancing	
Cycling outdoors	Handball		
Stationary bicycling	Racquetball		
Rowing			
Mini-trampoline			
Stair climbing			
Aerobic dancing			

cises that fit the aerobic definition and a list of nonaerobic exercises that are either too "stop and go," too short in duration, or too low in intensity.

There seems to be something magical about doing twelve minutes of an aerobic exercise. In fact, we can't even classify an exercise as aerobic unless it lasts for a minimum of twelve minutes — nonstop. Two six-minute exercises don't add up to one twelve-minute exercise. I don't mean that shorter exercises are worthless; I mean that they are less efficient at producing the heart and muscle enzyme changes that are so valuable in altering our metabolism. Some exercises require more time to achieve the same effect because during the first few minutes your heart rate hasn't reached its training zone. (Training zone is discussed in Chapter 11.)

In the table on page 33, several of the best aerobic exercises have been separated into three categories based on this principle. If you choose an exercise from Category II, which has a fifteen-minute minimum time, it will take your heart about three minutes to reach the training zone. If you choose an exercise from Category III, it will take about eight minutes to reach your training rate. In effect, one must tack on warm-up time to the twelve minutes of exercise.

Aerobic Exercises

I *Required minimum time 12 minutes*	II *Required minimum time 15 minutes*	III *Required minimum time 20 minutes*
Jumping rope	Jogging	Outdoor bicycling
Jumping jacks	Running	Stationary bicycling
Chair stepping	Dancing	Ice skating
Cross-country skiing	Mini-trampoline	Roller skating
Rowing		Swimming

If you find that when you run (a Category II exercise), it takes only one minute for your heart to reach its training zone, theoretically you could finish your exercise in thirteen minutes. I advise against this, however. Do not try to warm up fast by running fast in the first few minutes. Conversely, if it takes your heart a longer time to reach the training rate, then you must exercise longer than the suggested time. The rule is, exercise twelve minutes in your training zone plus however long it takes your heart to reach that training zone. It is difficult to determine this on your own, so I urge you to stick to the chart.

The next logical question is, if twelve minutes at the training heart rate is good, wouldn't twenty-four minutes be better? The answer is definitely yes. But the first twelve minutes produce a much more lasting effect than the second twelve minutes. We urge people to exercise longer than twelve minutes if they wish, knowing that their improvement will be faster. We must admit, however, that you get less and less for your effort beyond twelve minutes. It's an example of the law of diminishing returns. For this reason we urge beginners to do twelve minutes of exercise six days a week rather than a thirty-minute exercise three days a week. People who are already quite fit may profit more from the latter. For them, extra long exercise may be the only way to reach a competition training level. But we don't suggest this for the other 98 percent of the population.

Please don't misinterpret my emphasis on exercise. I do *not* mean that each daily exercise burns up lots of calories. Jogging for twenty minutes, for example, consumes only 180 calories, approximately the caloric content of a glass of milk. You would have to jog for days to use up the calories in a hot fudge sundae. Many studies in the literature support the point that each minute of exercise uses few calories. But we use calories when we are *not* exercising, even when we are asleep, and the exercised body seems to use more calories.

Furthermore, such studies overlook the long-term cumulative effects. It is ridiculous to expect reversal of muscle enzyme loss and of fatty infiltration of muscle in such short periods. Such changes take many months, or even years in very fat people.

The point of this chapter is that proper exercise changes muscle, which in turn alters the body's use of calories. It is a simple fact that those who exercise aerobically on a regular schedule do not get fat. If I were offering a pill to decrease the tendency of the body to make fat, fat people would be lining up to buy it. I AM OFFERING SUCH A PILL; IT TAKES JUST TWELVE MINUTES A DAY TO SWALLOW IT!

9

How Hard Should I Exercise?

THE INFORMATION in this chapter includes some very large changes since *Fit or Fat?* was first published in 1977. The first change is that my original emphasis on exercising at 80 percent of your maximum heart rate has been modified by research indicating that a great many metabolic changes can be brought about by exercising at lower intensities. We now urge a range of 65–80 percent of maximum heart rate rather than a fixed 80 percent. It's obvious that a training *range* is a whole lot easier to work with than an absolute number. It allows you to vary the intensity and duration of your workout to meet specific needs. If you're in a hurry, for instance, you can exercise at a higher intensity in the upper end of the range for a shorter time and still get a good aerobic, fat-decreasing workout. On the other hand, you can slow down and exercise longer for the same benefits. *If you stay in the training zone,* a long, gentle workout is just as effective as a shorter, more intense one.

In some cases lower intensities are mandatory! For example, older people's bodies repair more slowly. If they exercise at 80 percent, their muscles may not recover completely in twenty-four hours. If they exercise at 80 percent every day, they may get less fit instead of fitter. The body improvement that we expect from exercise depends on tissue repair, that is, protein being built into new tissue. Since age slows down this process, older people should either wait longer between exercise periods or exercise at lower intensities so there isn't as much stress on their tissues.

General systemic illness can also slow down healing and growth of new tissue. Suppose you had a mild case of mononucleosis, but you exercised every day at 80 percent of your maximum heart rate. You might find it harder and harder to exercise instead of easier. Your body would be trying to tell you, "I can't combat this mononucleosis and build new muscle at the same time." On the other hand, exercise at 65 percent of your maximum heart rate might allow your body to fight the mono and also build a little bit of improvement into your fitness mechanisms.

The same principle holds true for people recovering from injury and for women who are pregnant. When your body needs to repair tissue in a broken arm or synthesize new tissue for a baby, making new enzymes so that you can run faster is not on its high-priority list. If you exercise at 80 percent of maximum while pregnant or injured, you may be asking for more than your body can do. It says, "Hey! I'm making baby John and repairing that bunged-up knee. I'm not about to give up the protein I need for these jobs." You don't see pregnant or injured animals trotting at their usual speeds, but you also don't see them sitting around. They just move more slowly.

Fat people also seem to do better with lower-intensity activity when they first start an exercise program. Fit people burn fat well at higher intensities of exercise, but fat people do not. Their fat-burning machinery needs to be tuned up with lots of low-intensity exercise before they "rev up" into higher gears. Instead of shooting for a minimum of twelve to fifteen minutes of exercise at 80 percent of maximum heart rate, fat people would profit far more from thirty to forty-five minutes at a slower pace.

Another time your body repairs slowly is when it is stressed. Actually, all of the examples I've given — illness, injury, pregnancy — are kinds of stress. Even a strict or severely unbalanced diet is stressful and results in more protein breakdown than protein repair. Emotional stress can be just as taxing as physical stress. People lose protein during the stress of a divorce or after the death of a loved one. If your body is stressed in any way, it would be silly to add the stress of high-intensity exercise. But! Mild, maintenance exercise has lots of value.

10

Why Twelve Minutes?

In *Fit or Fat?* I emphasized that to be aerobic, an exercise must last a minimum of twelve minutes. Since then, however, people have pointed out that in subsequent publications and in my lectures, I have said fifteen minutes, twenty minutes, and sometimes forty minutes. To add to the confusion, many other authors push for thirty minutes. Who's right?

In a sense, we all are. Let's look at the purpose of exercise so that we can understand why there are so many different opinions on how long we should do it. WE EXERCISE TO CHANGE MUSCLE CHEMISTRY SO THAT WE WILL BURN FAT MORE EFFICIENTLY.

Many people mistakenly believe that it takes twelve minutes of aerobic exercise before fat is burned. They think their muscles use glucose for twelve minutes and then start using fat. This is incorrect. Fat is burned from the very start of the exercise. The only time fat isn't used is when you're exercising too hard for the fat-burning enzymes to function. (See Chapters 11 and 12 to make sure you understand how hard you should exercise.)

The question is, if fat is burned from the very start of exercise, what difference does it make how long we exercise? Why do I emphasize a minimum time of twelve minutes? The answer is that you are trying to produce *growth* of fat-burning enzymes, and a minimum of twelve minutes of continual, gentle activity seems to be the time trigger necessary to stimulate this growth.

Before I continue, please be sure you understand the difference between actual fat burning and growth of fat-burning enzymes. That's like the difference between burning logs in a fireplace and building a fireplace to burn logs. If you are fat, you have a little tiny fireplace that can burn only a few fat logs. Twelve minutes of aerobics helps you to build, over months, a bigger fireplace that can burn many fat logs. While you DO burn fat during aerobic activity, the growth of fat-burning enzymes is the real purpose for exercising. You want more and more "butter-burning" enzymes so that a year from now a greater proportion of the calories you use up during exercise are fat calories instead of sugar (glucose) calories. You want more fat-burning enzymes so that a year from now your body is a fat-*burning* machine instead of a fat-*storing* machine. You want a body that burns fat easily even when you don't exercise.

The minimum amount of exercise time required to increase those enzymes depends on how much muscle you use. The more muscle used, the less time you need to spend exercising. If you wiggle your fingers hard and vigorously for thirty minutes a day, you can't expect much change in your whole body. The amount of muscle involved is so small that your heart, lungs, and fat-burning machinery will hardly notice it. If finger wiggling were aerobic, there wouldn't be any fat piano players. It's not until you start using the big muscles in the lower body that you get a whole-body systemic effect.

As more and more muscle is incorporated into an exercise, less and less time is needed to stimulate enzyme growth. The key to this issue is the *proportion* of muscle used with respect to total body weight. There are lots of muscles in the upper body, but an upper-body exercise is not quite aerobic because the proportion of muscles used in comparison to total body weight is small.

Having established that the muscles in the lower body must be used for an exercise to be aerobic, let's look at why different exercises require different minimum times to stimulate enzyme growth. Think of an exercise that uses the muscles of the lower body only. Stationary bicycling immediately comes to mind. It's mainly leg work with perhaps a small amount of buttock work. Using that much muscle will spark a systemic response, but it will take about eight minutes for this response to begin, as evidenced by the slower rise in heart rate and slower increase in breathing. Once the systemic response is achieved, THEN you start counting your twelve minutes. In effect, twenty minutes of stationary bicycling yields twelve minutes of aerobic exercise and eight minutes of warming up.

More muscle is called into use when you start jogging. Now you're pumping your arms a bit, there's spring to your stride, and even muscles you don't think about, such as the chest muscles, are contributing to the overall effort. It seems that about fifteen minutes of jogging is all that's needed to produce the same aerobic results as twenty minutes of stationary bicycling. If you start doing something really vigorous, such as cross-country skiing, practically every muscle in your body is being used, and the required minimum time to elicit an aerobic response drops to twelve or thirteen minutes. The rise in heart rate and breathing is almost instantaneous, meaning that the systemic response is also nearly instantaneous.

Walking is an incredibly easy, efficient movement requiring very little muscle. Very sick people can walk. People with many broken bones have walked away from car accidents. I'm not talking about backpacking, mountain hiking, power walking, or race walking. I am talking about just plain, level walking. It doesn't require much muscle. Thirty or even forty minutes of steady walking is probably required to get aerobic benefits.

You can now see that every aerobic exercise needs to last a minimum of twelve minutes. Then, depending on how much musculature is used and therefore how much warm-up time is needed before a systemic response begins, you need to add on extra minutes. The Category I, II, and III exercises listed in Chapter 8 should be used only as guidelines. As you become more proficient at determining your appropriate exercise intensity by monitoring your breathing and heart rate (described in Chapters 11 and 12) you'll automatically know when you're exercising aerobically and at what point you can start the twelve-minute countdown.

AEROBIC EXERCISE

A. Is steady, nonstop.
B. Lasts twelve minutes minimum.
C. Has a comfortable pace.
D. Uses the muscles of the lower body.

11

How Do I Know If I'm in the Training Zone?

BY NOW YOU'RE probably saying, "Okay, I understand that there's a range of exercise intensities and that under some circumstances I may benefit more if I exercise at the low end of the range. But how do I know if I'm in the range?"

Here is another major change from my original book in 1977. At that time, the intensity of exercise was largely based on the formula *220 minus your age = maximum heart rate.*

In those days we thought that this formula applied to a large percentage of the population, as much as 86 percent. We now know it applies to only about 60 percent. Approximately 15 percent of the population have hearts that beat considerably slower than the predicted maximum and another 15 percent have hearts that beat much faster. This doesn't mean there's anything wrong with these hearts or that they are abnormal. It just means they aren't *average.*

Let's say your heart beats faster than average during exercise. If you're thirty years old, you would expect your heart to beat 220 minus 30, or 190 beats a minute when you exercise at maximum. But yours goes 210. It's as if you have a Kawasaki heart: it's built very well but it's made to function at a high RPM. When you exercise, your heart goes much faster than all the charts say it should, and your aerobics instructor is afraid you're going to die any minute. You're not — you just have a heart that beats very fast and is therefore off the chart.

Another 10 percent of the population (I'm only guessing at this number) is taking medication that affects heart rate. These people's hearts may fit the predicted formula, but the medication artificially depresses their heart rate during exercise. Pulse monitoring as a measure of exercise intensity is not reliable for this group either.

If you add together the 15 percent of people with slow-beating hearts, the 15 percent with fast-beating hearts, and the approximately 10 percent on some kind of medication, you have 40 percent of the population for which the 220 minus age formula becomes completely useless. Only about 60 percent of the population finds the formula to be a useful one.

Before I discuss the heart-monitoring approach to exercise, let me tell you a newer method. The new approach is simply to use common sense. When you are doing aerobic exercise, keep in mind the basic intention of the exercise. You're not trying to burn a lot of calories. You're saying to your body, "Please adapt to this so that tomorrow I can exercise better than I did today."

What you are really after is an adaptation phenomenon, since the body seems to adapt to whatever treatment it receives. It adapts to hard, intense exercise by changing muscles so that they burn sugar well and fat poorly. Slow, gentle exercise, on the other hand, turns muscles into fat-burning machines. It's the time you spend urging your body to change that really matters. The body adapts beautifully to steady pressure, just as teeth can be moved by the gentle, steady pressure of braces. I see men who run like crazy around the local track, proud that they can cover a mile in six minutes flat, and then wonder why they still must fight a bulging waistline. Such exertions are as effective in weight control as trying to move teeth with a hammer. Run slower and longer and let your body adjust.

With this in mind, you need to adjust the intensity of your exercise; your pace should be comfortable enough that you can continue beyond the minimum twelve minutes without feeling fatigued. You should be breathing deeply but not gasping. Some people call this the "perceived level of exertion," while others simply use what they call the "talk test." Say you are jogging with a friend. Is he able to talk, but you are not? Each of you should be able to talk a little bit, but neither of you should be able to sing an aria. For fun, try singing "God Bless America." If you can't get beyond the first word without gasping, you're exercising too hard. On the other hand, if you get past "land that I love" before you need your first breath, you should speed up.

When I'm teaching people how to exercise, I use the "talk to me" test. It's the same basic idea. If you're on a stationary bicycle, I say, "Can you talk to me? What's your name? Where do you live? What's your phone number?" If you can't talk to me without huffing and puffing and groaning, I know that the bicycle tension is too tight or you're pedaling too fast. Either one means you are doing *an*aerobic exercise. Your muscles are working without oxygen.

Exercising according to your perceived level of exertion or by using the talk test just boils down to using common sense. As you exercise, think to yourself, "Am I doing something so gentle and easy that I can go on for twenty, twenty-five, thirty minutes? Will my body change tonight as a result of this, or am I exercising too slowly or too fast?" If you are able to talk haltingly and are breathing deeply but comfortably, then you are almost certainly within the training zone. There's nothing wrong with occasionally exercising outside your training zone, but it doesn't fit the definition of aerobics.

Once you have found a comfortable exercise intensity, try taking your pulse. For 60 percent of you, the pulse you get should be between 65 and 80 percent of the formula 220 minus your age (maximum heart rate). But maybe you belong in the other 40 percent. Stick with the comfortable, common-sense intensity. We would probably find that the heart rate you get while exercising at that comfortable rate is 65 to 80 percent of your true under-lying maximum heart rate as determined on a treadmill.

Even though it doesn't fit everyone, we still recommend heart-rate monitoring of exercise as a useful tool. Having presented these two new pieces of information, first, that the formula 220 minus your age doesn't fit all people and, second, that exercising at low levels is far, far more beneficial than we originally thought, let's take a look at exactly how pulse monitoring works.

12

Heart-Rate-Monitored Exercise

LET'S TURN NOW to those people whose hearts do not beat unusually fast or unusually slow during exercise and who aren't taking medication that affects the heart rate. Let's just talk about average people, approximately 60 percent of the population. That 60 percent can make good use of pulse monitoring during and after exercise to judge the intensity of their exercise.

Recommended Heart Rates During Exercise*

Age	Maximum heart rate	85% of max. (athlete training rate)	65–80% of max. (recommended training range)	65% of max. (heart disease history)
				Not to exceed
20	200	170	130–160	130
25	195	166	127–156	127
30	190	162	124–152	124
35	185	157	120–148	120
40	180	153	117–144	117
45	175	149	114–140	114
50	170	145	111–136	111
55	165	140	107–132	107
60	160	136	104–128	104
65 +	150	128	98–120	98

*Based on resting heart rate of 72 for males and 80 for females. Men over forty and people with any heart problem should have a stress electrocardiogram before starting an exercise program.

As indicated in the table, your heart rate typically reaches a maximum for your age, and it will not beat any faster no matter how much harder you exercise. For young people, twenty years or under, this maximum is about 200 beats a minute. A forty-year-old person's heart has a maximum of 180 beats a minute.

You might think that a well-trained athlete would have a higher maximum pulse than someone who isn't physically fit. Not so. You might also think that women would have higher maximum pulses than men since they are generally smaller. But there are only slight differences between the maximums for men and women.

For regular, everyday, efficient exercise you should work only hard enough to make your heart go at 65–80 percent of the maximum for your age. If you are forty, your maximum heart rate should be 180, and you should exercise hard enough to get your heart going no more than 80 percent of that maximum: 80 percent of 180 equals 144 beats per minute.

Let's consider three forty-year-old men. The first is terribly out of shape, which means he has a lot of intramuscular fat as well as some obvious subcutaneous fat bulging under his skin. He might easily drive his pulse to 144 by just walking briskly. A second man, in better shape, might have to jog to get 144 beats per minute. And a third forty-year-old, lean and athletic, might have to run quite a fast pace to reach the same heart rate. You may think that the third man is getting the most exercise, while the first man is being quite lazy. But in fact they are all exercising equally, getting the same heart, lung, and muscular benefits.

For years the fat man who has tried to jog with his trim friend has felt he must jog at the same speed to get the same exercise. Now he can see that he should walk, jog, or run at whatever speed gives him the correct heart rate.

Husbands who are athletic are often guilty of pushing their wives into too strenuous exercise. They coerce their wives into going out for "just a little jog together." He runs slower for her and she runs faster for him. One is underexercised, the other is overexercised, and it is inefficient exercise for both of them. Men and women should think twice about exercising together because of the difference in their muscle mass. The average man has 20 percent more muscle than the average woman and 30 percent less fat.

If the man is several years older than the woman, or if he is quite out of condition and the woman is in good condition, then "coed" running seems to work well. Otherwise, women will get more benefit from their exercise if they slow down and exercise alone or with another woman.

Never again let anyone push you into exercising at his rate. Just take a look at the heart rate table on page 46 to determine the correct exercise training zone for you. Then pick any one of the steady aerobic exercises listed, or for that matter, any steady exercise. Do that exercise, in that range, for at least twelve minutes nonstop six days per week. The first few times you should stop after a minute or two to take your pulse. If the pulse is lower than your correct training zone, you aren't exercising hard enough. If the pulse is too high, just slow down a bit. Taking your own pulse like this is called "pulse-monitored exercise." It's as if you were being watched over by the world's best coach.

Here are a few pointers on taking your pulse. You'll need a watch or clock with a sweep-second hand. You can find your pulse on the thumb side of your wrist. Sometimes it's difficult to find the pulse in the wrists of women or older people, so try the side of your neck also. Lay your fingertips against the side of your neck. One of your fingers will pick up the pulse. Don't take your pulse with your thumb. It has its own pulse, and you might get a double count. Once you have found the pulse, count it for exactly 6 seconds. Multiply the number of beats you counted by 10. Most people get a count of 60, 70, 80, or 90. Take your pulse again, and this time be careful to note whether you were between numbers at the end of 6 seconds. You should get good enough at 6-second pulses to count half beats or even quarter beats. For example, suppose you count your pulse as "One, two, three, four, five, six, and one-half." That's a pulse of 65.

This is your resting pulse. You should take your pulse several times during the day to get your *average* resting pulse. As I mentioned earlier, most women average about 80 beats a minute and men about 72 beats a minute. Here is that word "average" again. It may be average to have a resting pulse of either 72 or 80, but it would be *normal* to have a much lower resting pulse. As you become more physically fit, your resting pulse drops. Very athletic individuals occasionally have a resting pulse as low as 35. Conversely, when you're ill and have a fever, the pulse rises sometimes to over 100 beats a minute.

I have a good friend who is a superathlete. Ed missed being in the Olympics in *three* different events. One time when we were camping, I decided to take Ed's pulse. At first I didn't think I had the right spot because I couldn't feel a beat. He tried to find it and also had trouble. Well, it turns out we didn't wait long enough. Ed had a resting pulse of 36! So I said, "Ed, what happens to your pulse when you exercise?" He didn't know, but he obligingly took off on a one-mile run through the woods, knocking down trees and brush that got in his way. He came lumbering back into the camp about seven minutes later, and I quickly took his pulse. It had gone all the way up to 39!

You have to picture the reserve this guy has. Every time his heart pumps, a gallon of blood must come out. When he exercises, his heart must be saying, "Ho-hum, I guess he wants me to pump more." And out comes another gallon. If you exercise correctly and long enough, the heart muscle will get stronger and will pump more slowly, pumping more blood with each stroke.

You may have reacted negatively to taking a pulse for such a short count. Members of the medical profession have been so indoctrinated with the fifteen-second pulse that they immediately assume a six-second pulse to be a layman's approach. I must admit that I reacted this way myself at first. But, if you want to measure your pulse during an exercise, it's usually necessary to stop the exercise momentarily. As you relax, naturally your heart starts to relax also, and your heart rate quickly slows down. If you count the pulse for the usual fifteen seconds, the count will be completely false because your heart will be beating faster at the beginning of the count and slower at the end. Furthermore, since the heart rate slows down more quickly as one gets in better condition, six-second pulses become more and more important the healthier one gets.

The only exercise I can think of in which you can take your training pulse without stopping the exercise is stationary bicycling. When you want to check your pulse rate with any other exercise, you'll have to stop and do a *quick* six-second count. (Remember, a fifteen-second pulse is not valid under these circumstances.) When you first start a new exercise you may have to stop several times to check your pulse until you know exactly how hard to do the exercise to get the correct rate. After that, you should be able to do the entire twelve minutes nonstop and only check it at the end.

I have cautioned you many times not to drive your pulse rate above the training zone. Be sure to check your training zone often. Many people find that after several weeks of the same exercise, their hearts don't reach the training zone. In most cases this simply means you should run faster, pedal with more resistance, jump higher, or what have you. And if this doesn't appeal to you, simply switching to a different exercise will often get your heart to its training zone.

I'm repeatedly asked if older people and those who are badly out of shape should "ease" into an exercise program. Isn't it too much for such people to start right out at twelve minutes a day? Certainly not! The whole point of aerobic exercise is that it prevents you from overexercising. If you are terribly out of shape, you may not even be able to walk briskly for the required period without getting out of breath. You need to decrease the *intensity* of your exercise, not the time spent doing it. I don't care if you have to crawl — do it for a full twelve minutes.

Gentle aerobic exercise, way below 80 percent of maximum heart rate, does far more good than we originally thought. Whether you pulse-monitor your exercise or use the talk test, use common sense. You aren't trying to burn a lot of calories or build a lot of muscle. You are asking your body to adapt to the exercise *after the exercise is over.* Ask your body to adapt just as an orthodontist moves teeth — gently.

13

The Stress EKG

HEART ATTACKS are so common in the United States and so disastrous that I can't pass up the chance for a few comments. There is no longer any question that regular aerobic exercise is a deterrent to heart attack. But once in a while someone drops dead of a heart attack while jogging — and he was jogging so he wouldn't have a heart attack! A few doctors use these isolated cases of heart attack during exercise as a reason for discouraging exercise. That's like saying we should do away with ambulances because they may have a wreck on the way to the hospital.

Still, people do have heart attacks while exercising, particularly if they exceed the comfortable pace I've been urging you to use. The best way to find out if you are at risk for a heart attack is to have a stress electrocardiogram (EKG). Most EKGs are taken with the person lying down and hence are no measure of possible abnormality during exercise. Such tests are called resting EKGs. The one you want is taken while you are moving.

Your car may run perfectly when it's idling but run poorly at high speed on the highway. So your mechanic has to race the engine during tune-ups to get an idea of how it's going to function at highway speeds. Similarly, if your doctor gives you a "complete" physical exam, including urinalysis, blood chemistry, and a resting EKG, and finds nothing wrong, all he can really say is, "You will be fine as long as you don't move."

To find out how the heart will function during exercise, the patient is asked to walk, then jog, then run on a treadmill while the heart is monitored by an EKG machine. A stress EKG will reliably indicate whether there is a possibility that you will have a heart attack during exercise. The speed of the treadmill is increased gradually so the intensity of the patient's effort increases gradually. The physician can stop the test at the first sign of abnormality rather than waiting for a heart attack.

The stress EKG is an excellent test to have before starting on an exercise program, particularly for men over forty and others in the high-risk group (those with a personal or family history of heart disease, high blood cholesterol, or long-term sedentary life style).

14

Aerobic or Anaerobic — What's the Difference?

MANY OF THE QUESTIONS that arise when one reads a book like this can be answered only by discussing the chemical reactions that take place in a muscle cell. There are whole books written on the subject with sleep-inducing titles like *Intermediary Metabolism* or *Physiological Chemistry*. Believe me, they don't make for pleasant Sunday afternoon reading. Nonetheless, I am going to try to give you a quick overview of the chemical reactions involved in a muscle cell as it attempts to extract energy from all that food we eat. Chemists will criticize me for oversimplification. But we can criticize them for making this important information so sticky that it isn't any fun. If you get bogged down reading it, just go on to the next chapters and come back to this one after your next aerobic exercise, when your brain cells are better oxygenated.

Glucose from carbohydrates, fatty acids from fats, and amino acids from proteins are burned inside muscle cells to get energy. But what does "burn" really mean in this context?

Burning in a muscle cell doesn't fit the image most of us have of burning. Let's pretend you have a small wooden building in your backyard that is no longer useful, so you decide to disassemble it and use its lumber for other projects. You have to do the job carefully, step by step, in order to avoid ruining each piece of lumber. It would be much simpler to touch a match to it and burn it down, except that you would have no lumber for your other projects. Cellular burning is like taking the building apart, a careful procedure requiring special tools called enzymes for each step, rather than burning it down.

It's important that you realize the significance of the enzymes involved. Literally hundreds of these fancy tools are needed in each cell, and each one is quite different from the others. Enzymes, which are made of protein, are large, complex molecules that cannot pass through the wall of a cell. Because the enzyme molecules are so large, it is folly to think that enzymes added to the diet or injected into the bloodstream will end up in muscle cells. The only way enzymes increase in a muscle is when DNA, the production manager of the cell, *makes* more enzymes inside the cell. This process is called enzyme biosynthesis, and it takes place only if you eat adequately, if your cells aren't sick, and if you exercise to stimulate the DNA to go to work.

Enzymes are delicate proteins. While all tissue proteins in the body are continuously breaking down and being repaired by DNA, the enzyme proteins break down the quickest. If you don't exercise, the DNA doesn't repair them as fast as they break down and your ability to burn calories decreases.

The burning (or disassembling) of glucose in a muscle cell takes place in two stages. During the first stage the glucose is broken down into pyruvic acid. In the second stage the pyruvic acid is completely disassembled into water and carbon dioxide, as shown in the diagram on page 56. The enzymes used during the first stage need very little oxygen to do their work. Hence this stage is referred to as the anaerobic phase (*an-* means "without"). The enzymes that function during the second stage need lots of oxygen, so this is called the aerobic phase.

We have defined aerobic exercise as exercise in which the heart rate is between 65 and 80 percent of maximum. In this training zone the heart and lungs are able to supply enough oxygen to the

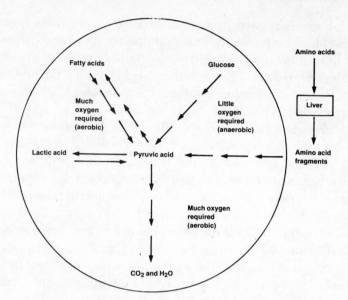

Energy Production Inside a Muscle

muscles so that glucose is disassembled through both stages and completely burned. If the exercise causes the pulse rate to exceed 80 percent of maximum, the heart and lungs cannot keep up with the oxygen demand in the muscle. When this happens, the glucose will only break down to pyruvic acid; there will not be enough oxygen to continue through the second stage. Exercise that exceeds 80 percent of maximum is called anaerobic exercise. Since pyruvic acid cannot be burned during anaerobic exercise, it accumulates in the muscle and is converted into lactic acid. Excess lactic acid in the muscle is painful. The pain is often so intense that you can't continue the exercise. When you stop and "catch your breath," oxygen flows into the deprived muscle. Most of the lactic acid turns back into pyruvic acid, to be burned aerobically. (It has been postulated that some of the remaining lactic acid is converted into fatty acids.)

A completely different set of enzymes is used for the burning of fats. Fatty acids, either from our fat deposits or from a recent meal, are carried by the blood to muscle cells. Inside the cell, the enzymes are lined up ready to take the fatty acid apart and get the energy out of it. Each enzyme does its work in an orderly sequence that biochemists call a chemical pathway. If you look at the diagram on page 56 you will see that the first half of fat burning (called the beta oxidation pathway) is unique to fats. The second half of fat burning uses the same enzymes as the second half of glucose burning.

Unlike glucose burning, in which the enzymes require little oxygen in the first stage, all the enzymes used in fat breakdown need a lot of oxygen. Anaerobic exercise, therefore, effectively shuts off all fat burning and forces the muscle to use glucose exclusively. The 65–80 percent maximum heart rate zone that I have been pushing not only allows you to burn fat while exercising, but also stimulates DNA synthesis of more of these enzymes. As the enzymes proliferate, you are better able to grab oxygen from the blood and to use fats at higher and higher exercise intensities. That is, you will be able to run faster, yet still run aerobically and burn increasing amounts of fat!

ANAEROBIC EXERCISE
builds sugar-burning enzymes.

AEROBIC EXERCISE
builds fat-burning enzymes.

Notice in the diagram that amino acids are also burned in muscle by the oxidative enzymes. This means that proteins can be burned along with fats and carbohydrates. Protein burning often occurs in people who are on very low calorie diets. The body can't get enough energy from fats or glucose and therefore burns valuable protein instead of using it for tissue repair.

Heavy weight lifting is at the extreme end of anaerobic exercise, whereas walking is perhaps at the extreme end of aerobic exercise. The trouble comes when we try to distinguish between exercises that are somewhere in the middle. For example, if I go out for a jog or a slow run, which type of exercise am I doing? The answer lies in whether I am running out of breath or not, whether I can continue on and on or have to stop. You should walk, jog, or run as fast as you can without getting out of breath, without feeling exhausted when you quit. Exercise that requires this sort of effort guarantees that your fat-burning enzymes are functioning, that they aren't shutting down because there's too little oxygen available.

Sometimes the breathing and talk test guidelines described in Chapter 11 don't work. If a person hates to exercise, he'll quit when he gets out of breath — "mentally." More often, however, the breathing and talk test doesn't work because the person won't slow down for anything. He won't admit he's out of breath.

This latter group of diehards, or jocks, are almost always men with an athletic past. They are the ones who overstress themselves to their own detriment and who break up their marriages by exhorting their wives, "Run faster, honey! Can't you keep up?!"

I have to admit to belonging to the jock group myself, and I will tell you an embarrassing tale to make a point. In graduate school at M.I.T. I played a lot of hard squash, and I was quite good at it. Squash, like racquetball and handball, is really a series of short anaerobic bursts. An hour of that game will exhaust almost anyone. So I thought I was in great shape. Once in a while I played with a dentist friend named Lou, who preferred to run but who enjoyed our occasional games of squash. I could usually beat him, but I was always surprised at how well he played and how long he could last despite playing so rarely. One day Lou talked me into going for a long, slow run with him. After about half a mile, I had to stop and vomit. I didn't seem to have any guts for it. Well, now I know what was going on. Lou's aerobic running got him in shape for my sport, but my anaerobic sport wasn't getting me in shape for his.

One of my main reasons for writing this chapter is to point out the importance of muscle enzymes, particularly the fat-burning enzymes. If you haven't got enzymes, you are going to get fat. Enzymes will increase only if you stimulate the DNA by exercise and by eating enough calories so that there will be amino acids available for biosynthesis.

15

If Two Aspirins Are Good, Four Must Be Better

NOTICE THAT the heart rate table on page 46 also contains an 85 percent column. Trained athletes, familiar with competition, can benefit from exercise of greater intensity. Although much of their training is between 65 and 80 percent of maximum, they occasionally push themselves to bouts of 85–95 percent of maximum. Please don't make the mistake of putting yourself in this column if you don't belong there. Men in particular are inclined to believe that if moderate exercise is good, intense exercise is better. But if your body isn't ready for it, you will overstress the muscles and do more damage than good. If you want fast improvement, you should exercise longer rather than harder.

When Hal walked into my clinic after a six-month absence, my jaw dropped. The man looked five years older and sick! I managed to hide my dismay because Hal was obviously elated. "I've lost twenty pounds in six months just from running," he said proudly. And it was true; Hal was thinner — to the point of gauntness. Something was seriously wrong. Sure enough, when he was tested for body fat, he had lost both fat *and* muscle!

Of the twenty pounds he had lost, seven and a half were muscle (see the table on page 61). That explained why he looked so hollow, why his skin seemed to hang. I thought for sure Hal had gone on some strange diet, but when questioned he insisted that it was only the running that had caused him to lose weight. Then it hit me! Hal must have been *over*exercising. We've already discussed that you lose muscle if you diet improperly. Loss of muscle also occurs if you overexercise!

And that is what had happened. Hal had decided that he wanted to get in shape really fast, so every day for six months he had run two miles with a heart rate of 160 beats per minute. This would have been a reasonable heart rate if Hal were twenty years old, but Hal was fifty. Every day for six months he had been driving his heart rate nearly 15 percent over the recommended rate. This was overstressing his muscles, and they weren't able to repair themselves.

Hal's Loss of Lean Mass Due to Overexercise

	Before	After
Total Weight	170 lbs.	150 lbs.
LBM	127.5 lbs.	120 lbs.
Fat	42.5 lbs.	30 lbs.
% Fat	25%	20%

Hal was overexercising in a second way. He was exercising too often with the same exercise. As you get older, it's a good idea to switch exercises from day to day. (For example, run on Monday, Wednesday, and Friday, and cycle on Tuesday, Thursday, and Saturday.) Muscles don't repair as quickly with age. By switching exercises, you give the set of muscles you stressed on Monday time to build up while you stress another set on Tuesday. By Wednesday the "Monday muscles" are not only repaired but also stronger than ever.

So poor Hal had put his muscles in double jeopardy. They were being overworked when he exercised and then he didn't give them time to repair between exercises. Eventually they gave up. The result was that Hal had seven and a half pounds less body machinery than when he started the program.

REMEMBER: IF YOU'RE IN A HURRY TO GET IN SHAPE, EXERCISE LONGER, NOT HARDER.

We had Hal change his exercise program. He now runs four miles twice a week and at a much slower pace, so that his heart never exceeds 140 beats per minute. And he now rides a stationary bicycle twice a week for about thirty minutes, again making sure that his heart rate stays at 140. When we saw Hal after another six-month interval he still weighed 150 pounds, but somehow he looked more rugged. And, of course, you know what had happened. The muscles were slowly building up. He still doesn't have as much muscle as he did originally, but with the fat content steadily decreasing and the muscle content increasing, I know he'll make it.

Hal's Improvement in Lean Body Mass

	Before	After incorrect exercise	After revised exercise
Total Weight	170 lbs.	150 lbs.	150 lbs.
LBM	127.5 lbs.	120 lbs.	123.7 lbs.
Fat	42.5 lbs.	30 lbs.	26.3 lbs.
% Fat	25%	20%	17.5%

16

Wind Sprints

I HOPE I have cautioned you as strongly as I possibly could in the previous chapters to monitor your aerobic exercise and to realize that slow aerobic exercise is often better than hard aerobic exercise. However, I don't want you to go away with the feeling that Covert Bailey says, "Never get out of breath. Never exercise anaerobically." That would not be true.

People involved in sports have a strong desire to become ever fitter. To increase aerobic fitness, it works well to occasionally and deliberately exercise so that you get out of breath, to go against all the warnings I have given you in the last chapters. I'm referring to interval training, more commonly known as wind sprints.

Basically a wind sprint consists of a very fast, very short exercise in the middle of your otherwise aerobic exercise. Suppose the aerobic exercise you like is jogging. You're jogging comfortably along a road out in the country, as you've done many times. You know how to jog along that road without getting out of breath. In the middle of your comfortable jog, do a short sprint. Run fast for a very short distance, something like a quarter the length of a football field, far enough to get out of breath. Sometimes I use the distance between telephone poles as a measure. When you slow down, return to the speed you were jogging at before. That original speed is now no longer comfortable because you are in oxygen debt after doing the anaerobic sprint. However, if you keep jogging at that pace, after four or five telephone poles or a few hundred yards, you eventually relieve your oxygen debt, and your breathing becomes comfortable again. Now, sprint again!

Wind sprints are THE fastest way to increase fitness. In essence, what you are doing is demanding that your body recover under stress. Many athletes mistakenly think that it is the wind sprint itself that raises fitness levels. Not so. Fitness is improved during the period *after* the sprint when your body is forced to recover while you continue to run.

We don't encourage wind sprints for people who are quite fat or who haven't exercised in a long time, because they tend to overdo it. Since they aren't familiar with the routine, their bodies hurt. They run too fast during the sprint and slow down too much during the recovery. They need to wait until they can exercise comfortably for at least thirty minutes before adding wind sprints to their program.

On the other hand, I don't think it's fair to my readers to overlook the fact that many of you are really quite fit, or at least you used to be; maybe now you have only ten or fifteen pounds to lose. You're used to exercise and are familiar with interval training. Even you, however, need to be cautioned about the real purpose of wind sprinting. Remember, the sprint itself does not induce change. It's the recovery period afterward, as you maintain your aerobic pace even though you're out of breath, that produces a change. For this reason, the speed and length of the wind sprint are not that important. You DON'T have to run as fast as possible. You DON'T have to sprint a great distance. You simply have to run fast enough and far enough to get out of breath.

We find that wind sprints work for lots of people. We've even had people who are very fat and very out of shape use them, but I caution you, I urge you, I *implore* you not to try them until you really know what your aerobic level is. After you have been doing gentle aerobic exercise for several months, your fitness level will probably reach a plateau, and occasional wind sprints will help to boost it. But it is pointless to start doing wind sprints if you haven't established a comfortable long-distance, long-time aerobic level. If you haven't been exercising long enough to know exactly what pace is comfortable for you, it would be foolish indeed to apply the theory of the wind sprint.

17

Choosing an Aerobic Exercise

I MEET MANY PEOPLE who are all fired up to begin an exercise program, only to give up after a few weeks. Inevitably, it turns out that they selected an exercise not suited for them or they overexercised, or both. I cannot caution you too often — be sure to exercise at the appropriate training zone and breathing intensity!

I remember with horror the story of Gina. She was fifty-three years old and had no history of exercise. But she heard me lecture and decided that running in place was going to be her exercise. When I saw her six months later, she told me she had given up after five days. She felt very guilty, but the exercise had made her so tired that she couldn't do anything for the rest of the day. When I asked her to describe what she had done, she said she had run in place for about four minutes and then had fallen on the couch, exhausted. She did that for five days and quit.

"What was your pulse rate?" I asked.

Well, she hadn't bothered to take it; it didn't seem important.

"How hard were you breathing?" I asked.

"I was gasping!"

So I had her demonstrate for me exactly what she had done. After running in place for one minute, sure enough, she was wheezing and heaving. I had her stop and took her pulse. It was 170 beats a minute! This was a woman whose recommended training range is 109–134 beats a minute. I nearly had a heart attack worrying if *she* was going to have a heart attack. After a few minutes of rest, I had her try again, but this time I had her lift her feet only about four inches off the floor. It was still too strenuous. This time her heart was beating at 152 and she was still panting much too hard. Finally, I had her run in place by simply lifting her heels, keeping her toes on the floor. This exercise was enough to keep her heart in the training range and allow her to breathe deeply but comfortably. To most of us this seems ridiculous, but Gina was so unconditioned that simply wiggling her knees was an aerobic exercise.

Many people comment that they get bored doing the same exercise day after day. I don't blame them. What I am encouraging is that you do *some* kind of aerobic exercise day after day. During the summer months you'll find me jogging on Monday, Wednesday, and Friday, swimming on Tuesday and Thursday, and taking long bicycle or canoe trips on the weekend. In the winter it's jogging or jumping rope during the week, depending on the weather, and cross-country skiing on the weekend. Each of these exercises will result in overall, systemic cardiovascular fitness and general fat loss. Additionally, by switching exercises one avoids overdeveloping some muscles at the expense of others.

A long-distance runner's body, for instance, will adapt to the constancy of his exercise. His upper body will tend to thin out considerably. As the muscles in his arms, shoulders, and chest become fat-free, they also tend to shrink a little. This does not mean that these muscles are out of condition. Muscle biopsy studies of these tissues show the extremely high enzyme counts indicative of aerobic fitness (see Chapter 14). Most runners will tell you that the sacrifice of upper body size is well worth the rewards, both mental and physical, of their sport. But if you dislike an unproportioned physique, doing a variety of exercises will tend to keep your musculature "evened out."

It's surprising how easily aerobic exercises are assimilated into

What about warming up and cooling down? In general, these both should be a "dress rehearsal" of your exercise. If you decide to jog, the best warm-up is a very slow jog. And the best cool-down is a fast walk. The same is true of all the exercises: just do a slower version of the exercise to warm up or cool down. For the average person who plans to exercise for fifteen to forty-five minutes at moderate intensity, five minutes for warming up and another five minutes for cooling down is sufficient. People who exercise very intensely or for very long periods need more warm-up and more cool-down. Warm muscles are less likely to tear (muscle strain), and periods of warming up and cooling down are kinder to the heart and lungs.

Although I feel that warming up is necessary, I'm ambivalent about stretching. A properly stretched muscle is certainly going to give more than an unstretched one, but an *improperly* stretched muscle may be more injury-prone than one that is never stretched. When you stretch, remember three basic rules:

1. Never stretch muscles that haven't been warmed up. Warm up first, THEN stretch.
2. Stretch slowly, don't bounce.
3. Never stretch to the point where you are uncomfortable. A stretch should last 20–45 seconds. A good rule of thumb is this: if you feel you could hold the stretch indefinitely without pain, then you are not overstretching.

one's life style. Most of them become more than an exercise. They become a sport. Daily walking or jogging conditions you for weekend mountain hiking. Daily cycling, indoors or out, primes you for weekend bike excursions in the country. There are canoe trips for the daily rower. And the camaraderie with fellow weekend runners should not be missed by the jogger. Nonaerobic exercises are pretty exclusive. It's hard to imagine a weight lifter packing a picnic lunch and going out with his girl to lift weights all day by a lovely stream. Golf? Tennis? They're great sports but not great exercise. Common sense tells you that twelve minutes of tennis or golf will hardly get you conditioned.

I'm going to discuss various aerobic exercises; you can choose one or two that are suited for you, but please don't be like Gina. Find an exercise that gives you the correct training range and save the more strenuous exercises for later.

Now! On to the exercises!

Note that for each exercise I have indicated its long-term fat-burning potential and the risk of injury. In most but not all cases, exercises that have high fat-burning potential carry a greater risk of injury. Any exercise that is weight-bearing, uses a lot of different muscle groups, and involves bouncing and jarring of joints is bound to have victims. Running, one of the fastest fat-burning exercises, is currently getting a bad name from the growing list of runners who sustain injuries. But a closer look at statistics reveals that the majority of these injuries occur in those who run more than thirty-five miles a week.

Back in the 1970s, when *Fit or Fat?* was first published, people were pretty pigheaded about exercise. They'd insist on doing the same exercise day after day, week after week until they either became totally bored and stopped exercising or were injured and had to drop out. People seem to be more sensible today, varying their exercise routine among three or four "favorites." Even the diehard runners are finding that "cross-training" improves their running performance. If you especially enjoy doing one of the exercises that has a higher risk of injury, that's fine. Just don't overdo it. You can see from the following list that you can add high-fat-burning but low-injury-risk activities to your program without sacrificing the quality of your workout.

The following list is mainly for beginners trying to decide which exercises are best for them. For this reason, I've added a "special applications" category for each exercise to highlight those that meet special needs.

OUTDOOR AEROBIC EXERCISES

Jogging/Running

Long-term fat-burning potential: high.
Injury risk: moderate for mileages under 35 per week; very high over
35 miles per week.
Special applications: young, relatively fit people; older people if they
have prior conditioning from a walking program.

By far the best-known aerobic exercise, jogging or running is one
of the easiest programs to start. The only equipment you need is
a pair of good running shoes. In general, most of you who
haven't been in a running program will be classified as joggers
(there's controversy about this, but as a general rule of thumb, if
it takes you more than eight minutes to run a mile, you're jogging).

The injury risk with jogging/running is mainly to joints and
ligaments and muscles of the lower body. If you're plagued with
knee, ankle, or lower back pain you can try varying the length
of your stride, your speed, or your foot strike (a heel-ball step
works best when running a mile in more than eight minutes).
Even occasionally changing your style — skipping, or running
sideways or backward — will sometimes help. Run on softer
surfaces such as wood chip trails, composition, or rubberized as-
phalt. DO NOT persist if the pain doesn't let up in a day or two.
Switch to another exercise and have a doctor check out the problem.

Walking

Long-term fat-burning potential: moderately low if total walking time
is 30 minutes or less or walking speed is slower than 15 minutes a
mile; moderate if more than 30 minutes or faster than 15 minutes
a mile; high for race walking.
Injury risk: low.

Special applications: beginning exercisers, very overweight people, people over fifty, during pregnancy, athletes recovering from injury or illness.

Walking is the easiest program to start. No special skill is required — you already know how to walk — and it's always ready when you are. You don't have to worry about gathering up exercise gear, getting out equipment, driving to a gym. All you have to do is walk out your front door. Bad weather? Shopping mall walking has become a popular early morning activity in many cities.

Walking must be fairly vigorous to give aerobic fat-burning benefits. Try to set a pace of at least a hundred steps a minute and less than twenty minutes a mile. You have to walk for about forty-five minutes to equal twenty minutes of jogging.

Sometimes an overweight or older person is embarrassed to jog but finds that walking doesn't drive his pulse up high enough. I solved this problem for Jane, a favorite aunt of mine. I got a small backpack and filled it with bags of sand. We experimented with different weights until we found how much she needed to carry during her walks to get the right pulse rate. Now Aunt Jane greets a neighbor while out on one of her jaunts with, "The backpack? I just returned from Europe, my dear. Simply everyone wears them there. Quite the thing, you know!"

Race, or power, walking is rapidly gaining popularity, and I heartily applaud its proponents. The vigorous arm swinging and the odd hip movement that makes the power walker resemble a frantic duck really chew up the calories. Many race walkers can outpace joggers. I believe that after we get past the laughter, power walking is going to be the choice exercise of the future, giving a better workout with half the jarring impact of running.

Cycling

Long-term fat-burning potential: moderate.
Injury risk: low from the sport itself but high if collisions and accidents are included.

Special applications: a great group or family sport; sometimes good
   for those with back problems (consult your physician) and for
   overweight or older people.

Cycling is the exercise you fall in love with! Because it uses fewer
muscles than running and because it is not weight-bearing, you'll
have to cycle about forty minutes to equal twenty minutes of jogging. But most people don't mind at all. Bicycling is usually a
joyful pastime rather than an exercise drudgery. Moreover, when
elite runners and cyclists are compared, cyclists, as a group, come
out looking fitter. This is because the low injury rate among cyclists allows them to spend more time in training than runners,
who spend proportionally less time in training and more time in
recovery.
   Cycling does have drawbacks. A good bicycle can be expensive. It may not be easy to find nonstop routes so you can maintain a steady exercise pulse. Cycling requires some balance if
you're new at it, and it's tricky learning to change gears so you
can go smoothly up and down hills. Try to maintain a steady
pace of about 70 revolutions a minute instead of bursts of pushing and coasting.
   Mountain biking is fast becoming a popular sport among
those who are burned out with traditional cycling. It combines
the rustic pleasures of the backwoods with a strenuous workout while avoiding the dangers of not-so-watchful automobile
drivers.

Swimming

Long-term fat-burning potential: low.
Injury risk: very low.
Special applications: people with arthritis or other joint problems,
   during pregnancy, people recovering from injury, older people.

Swimming is the most injury-free sport around. It gives excellent
cardiovascular benefits and is great for toning practically all the
muscles of the body. But if you're overfat, I don't recommend it

as your only exercise. Of the thousands of people I've tested for body fat, swimmers consistently carry more fat than runners or cyclists.

Mammals that spend a lot of time in the water tend to conserve fat. Look at whales and seals. Both are very fit but very blubbery mammals. Human mammals that exercise frequently in water are like seals. The extra fat seems to be needed for warmth and buoyancy. Most of the fat in swimmers is subcutaneous rather than in the muscles. A swimmer's muscles are probably every bit as lean and fit as a runner's; it's just that their bodies adapt to a cold liquid environment by carrying fat under the skin.

So! You can get very fit with swimming, but you probably won't lose much fat. Please note that I have not said swimming makes you fat. When the original *Fit or Fat?* was published, quite a few swimmers were unhappy and angry over my remarks. They thought I was slandering their sport, when all I was doing was observing a natural body adaptation. While swimming usually does not decrease body fat, I have not said swimming will *add* fat. If you are 35 percent fat to start with, you will lose fat more slowly with swimming than with land sports. You will NOT get fatter. If you are lean and fit when you take up swimming, you will stay lean and fit. But your body fat will probably not decrease.

Despite this drawback, I think swimming is a good starting program for fat people who are unused to exercise. They can learn body coordination and gain fitness without feeling clumsy or risking injury to already overburdened joints. Once they've built up a certain amount of coordination and fitness, they can venture on to exercises that burn more fat.

Swimming requires a lot of practice before you're good enough at it to get a workout, and sometimes it's hard to commandeer a lane for laps. The novice ought to look into aqua-aerobics classes as an alternative. They're much more fun than boring lap swimming. Exercising against the water's resistance strengthens muscles without bumping and jarring. The buoyancy of the water buffers fast, jerky, potentially injury-inducing motions. Since most of the workout is in the shallow end, even nonswimmers can join in. Because aqua-aerobics classes are so new and every instructor has a different format, there's not much data available at this time regarding their effectiveness for increasing fitness and decreasing fat. But they're fun and certainly a good beginning exercise for older, fat, pregnant, or arthritic people.

Cross-Country Skiing

Long-term fat-burning potential: very high.
Injury risk: low.
Special applications: people who are already moderately fit.

The king of aerobic exercises! Cross-country skiing is the fastest fat burner, is more strenuous than running, yet has a low risk of injury because its movements are gliding rather than bouncing. The start-up costs are fairly low (compared to downhill skiing), or you can experiment with rental equipment. I recommend cross-country skiing for people who are already in pretty good shape. It's a deceptive exercise in that it requires skill and balance along with good arm and leg coordination. You'll be surprised how tiring it can be, even though your pace is usually slower than your jogging/running pace.

Cross-country skiing is no longer seasonal. There are several fine machines on the market that simulate the striding leg motion synchronized with arm and shoulder movement. There are also special ski skates available to help you stay in shape during summer months. Put rubber tips on your ski poles and "exer-stride" along your jogging trail.

INDOOR AEROBIC EXERCISES

Please try to find at least one indoor exercise for times when the weather is bad, or your time is limited, or small children prevent you from going outdoors. I like to use indoor exercise equipment as an adjunct to outdoor activity. Manufacturers claim that their devices are just as good as the real thing, but you just don't learn coordination and body sense from a stationary bicycle or a rowing machine. A machine is perfectly fine for getting fit, but there's something about stumbling and falling now and then that separates the athlete, the lover of sports, from the person who uses machines.

Many of the following exercises require the purchase of equipment. As a general rule of thumb, the heavier and more costly the machine, the better it is. If you get something cheap, it will probably end up as a fancy flower pot holder in six months. It's best to try the equipment before purchasing. Don't buy mail order equipment unless you've had a chance to use a friend's machine from that company. They usually come in hundreds of pieces you have to assemble, and if you find you don't like the machine, it's a hassle to return it.

Stationary Bicycling

Long-term fat-burning potential: moderate.
Injury risk: low.
Special applications: older people, people with joint problems, those who are overweight, during pregnancy, beginning exercisers.

Stationary bicycling is a good safe aerobic exercise. It doesn't require the balance and coordination necessary for outdoor cycling. It works well to maintain fitness during recuperation from ankle, foot, or thigh injuries. But, as most people complain, it's boring! Actually, I like stationary bicycling because I can do two things at once. While I'm exercising I can read a book or watch the evening news. There are bike videos available for those of you who prefer a scenic route during your indoor exercise. You can even try weight lifting while using a stationary bicycle. You can pedal while pumping small weights overhead to strengthen shoulders, do biceps curls, triceps back extensions, and frontal flies for the pectorals. And it's a great opportunity to get in shape while your fingernail polish is drying!

Rowing

Long-term fat-burning potential: high.
Injury risk: low.
Special applications: people who want to build upper-body muscle along with aerobic fitness, exercisers with an injured leg.

Indoors or outdoors, rowing is a high fat-consuming exercise. Like cross-country skiing, it exercises most of the large muscle groups without stress on joints and has the added benefit of developing the muscles of the upper torso. It's one of the few aerobic exercises that can be performed with one leg if you have an injury to the other.

Stair Climbing, Chair Stepping, Bench Stepping

Long-term fat-burning potential: high.
Injury risk: moderately low.
Special applications: easy for beginners, overweight people, during pregnancy.

Way back when exercise testing was in its infancy, the chair-step test used to be the standard method for determining fitness. It was simple. You got an eight-inch-high stool, stepped up with the right foot, brought the left foot up, stepped down with the right foot, then brought the left foot down. If you did this for fifteen minutes, you chalked up a fat-burning, cardiovascular-improving aerobic exercise for the day. This simple little exercise has now reaped millions of dollars for the manufacturers of stair-climbing machines.

The popularity of these machines is amazing. People have to make reservations days in advance to use one. Although they won't make you any more fit than climbing regular stairs, they

do offer some pluses, such as continuous uphill work and free-
dom from the concern you'd have exercising in a deserted, potentially dangerous, stairwell.

Bench-stepping classes have also become very popular. Each
person has a bench 1½ feet wide by 3 feet long and ranging in
height from 4 to 12 inches. You are led through a series of stepping combinations up, down, and around the bench. The ca-
dence is usually slower than regular aerobic dance classes, and
the easy routines are appealing to those frustrated with the more
intricate steps used in aerobic dance classes. Yet this seemingly
mild, low-impact exercise yields terrific fat-burning results. It's as
energy demanding as running but with no more force to the
joints than walking.

Jumping Rope

Long-term fat-burning potential: high.
Injury risk: moderately high.
Special applications: moderately fit people as a second exercise.

I think everyone should have a jump rope around "just in case."
If you're a runner, it's great to use when you're traveling and prefer not to run in strange neighborhoods. You could keep a jump
rope at work and use it instead of taking a fifteen-minute coffee
break. I've even jumped rope up and down the aisle of a 747
during a long overseas flight!

Jumping rope is best as an alternative exercise for those days
when time is limited or you'd rather stay indoors. It's a bit too
strenuous and hard on joints to be used every day.

Treadmill

Long-term fat-burning potential: moderate to high, depending on
incline and speed.
Injury risk: low.

Special applications: good for everyone; very fit people can steepen
   the incline or increase the speed for a good workout, while
   beginners or overweight people can use slower speeds and level
   walking.

The treadmill is a fine piece of equipment found in many health
clubs. Of simple design, it is a self-powered or motorized device
consisting of a slanted board on rollers with side bars for balance. By changing the incline or the speed, you can power walk,
run, or hike uphill. Many people find that they avoid the sore
knees and back problems associated with jogging when they
switch to a treadmill.

   Your best pace on a treadmill is a fast walk or slow jog. Unfortunately, the macho instinct emerges, and I've seen many overweight and unconditioned men running at a pace that even a seasoned runner would find difficult to maintain. Use some sense
with this machine. Go fifteen steady fat-burning minutes at a
moderate pace instead of three panting anaerobic minutes of
heart-stopping hell that you call "warming up."

Mini-Trampoline

Long-term fat-burning potential: moderately low.
Injury risk: low unless you bounce off the trampoline.
Special applications: beginners, people with joint problems, older
   people.

A mini-trampoline is a good piece of home equipment for those
just starting out in an exercise program. For the already fit, it
may not provide enough of a workout. You can vary your regular bouncing by running in place on it, jumping rope on it, or
dancing to music on it.

   I once lectured to an organization that had several of these
trampolines in the back of the room. When people in the audi-
ence wanted a break, they didn't go out for a smoke; instead,
they would go to one of the mini-trampolines. I could see heads

bobbing up and down as I continued the lecture. I thought this would be a distraction, but no one complained. As each person finished, he would quietly be replaced by another. This went on throughout the day and was one of the healthiest things I've ever seen.

Aerobic Dancing

Long-term fat-burning potential: high.
Injury risk: high in high-impact classes, low in low-impact classes.
Special applications: moderately fit women AND men.

Because aerobic dancing uses both upper and lower body musculature, you'll burn as much or more fat as you would in running. The classes use a variety of foot movements, so you reduce the risk of repetition-induced trauma. And because they're just plain fun, the "sticking with it" potential is far greater than with most other aerobic sports.

Although instructors vary their routines to avoid both boredom and injury, the vigorous jumping, weaving, and bouncing of aerobic dance classes still result in lots of twisted ankles, sore knees, and aching backs. The high injury rate has led to a trend in the last few years toward "low-impact" routines. In a low-

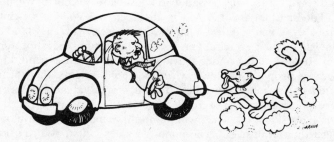

*Running your dog on a leash out the car
window is great exercise — for the dog.*

Will Hand-Held Weights Improve My Fitness?

Will holding weights during your walk, jog, or aerobic dance class make you fitter? Manufacturers of hand weights claim that you burn 50 percent more calories if you use them while exercising. This claim intrigued exercise physiologists, who promptly took the weights to their laboratories to see if it was true. So far, not one laboratory has been able to validate the claim. The most they can determine is that hand-held weights increase calorie expenditure 6–7 percent, which can be equaled by extending your exercise time by one or two minutes. The only time the weights seem to significantly increase calorie expenditure is when they are vigorously pumped overhead. You could do this during an aerobics class, but you'd have to be pretty gutsy to pull it off on the jogging trail without looking silly.

But it isn't the number of calories you burn that makes you more or less fit. Do hand-held weights do other things that might contribute to better fitness? Yes and no. The guys in the laboratory found that holding weights during exercise interfered with normal body movement, which may possibly make you more injury-prone. (If you swing the weight too vigorously, you might throw a shoulder out of joint.) Moreover, in people with a tendency toward high blood pressure, hand weights may exacerbate their problem. The conclusion of the physiologists seems to be that you can benefit just as much by exercising a little longer, so why take unnecessary risks with hand-held weights?

But wait a minute! Suppose you don't have high blood pressure and you are a sensible person who knows how to control weights and doesn't fling them loosely in all directions? Will you benefit? Probably. When people use hand weights SENSIBLY, they tend to slow down their exercise. This is one of the reasons the laboratory physiologists didn't notice a great increase in calorie expenditure. Because people slow down when they hold weights, their heart rate doesn't change very much. Instead, more total musculature is incorporated into the exercise. It's as if the heart says, "Because you have slowed down, I will pump the same amount of blood but to more muscles." The bonus to you is, first, you're using more muscle and, second, the slower speed reduces the risk of injury to the lower body.

impact class one foot is always touching the ground. There's no jumping up and down or sudden, jerky movements. To get the same workout as a high-impact class, participants do more upper-body exercise, sometimes using hand weights. Reliance on strong leg movements like high knee lifts, lunges, leg kicks, and multidirectional traveling (back and forth across the room) keep the energy expenditure high. Even the high-impact classes have been modified for those who still prefer to jump and whose bodies are strong enough to handle it. More emphasis is placed on bending the knees to minimize stress and landing on the ball of the foot first, then rolling onto the heel.

An added bonus included in most aerobic classes is muscle-building floorwork along with stretching and relaxation segments.

How to Get Started

▶ **Memorize these rules:**

1. Aerobic exercise has to involve the legs and the buttocks because we need to use the big muscles in the body to get a whole-body, systemic response.
2. It has to continue nonstop to be truly aerobic. You can't just walk down the street pausing to talk to everybody.
3. You should not get out of breath while you do it.

If you aren't following all three of these rules, then you aren't doing aerobic exercise.

▶ **If you can't do it right, do it often.**

What do I mean by this strange statement? People sometimes get *too* hung up on rules. They overlook the fact that a whole lot of "not quite aerobic" exercise can be just as good as a moderate amount of true aerobic exercise. Even though you may be breaking one of the three rules, you can still get aerobic benefit if you do a lot of it. For instance, the rule that you can't pause in the middle of your exercise would classify tennis as nonaerobic because it's a stop-and-go exercise. Nonetheless, if you play tennis for an hour or two, you can definitely increase aerobic fitness. Your body changes just as if you had been jogging nonstop.

Remember! If you can't exercise exactly by the rules I've given you, just do a lot of it. Quantity can substitute for quality. That's why sports sometimes makes people fitter than strict exercise at a health club.

▶ Don't exercise with a fit friend.

You probably can see the point of this one right off. If you are really fat or really out of shape, it's too hard on your body to run or bicycle at your fit friend's pace. Obviously, you can exercise with a fit friend if he or she is sensible and isn't trying to push you or make you feel bad. I'm only saying you should be careful. Sometimes, with the best intentions, fit friends push us too fast, too often, or too hard because it's so easy for them. We end up getting injured while they think the exercise was nothing.

▶ Start so slowly that people make fun of you.

I deliberately said that in a peculiar way so you'd pay attention. In the last ten to fifteen years we've learned a lot about the benefits of exercising more slowly than what we used to recommend. It needs to be emphasized over and over: gentle exercise pays off. If you are exercising at a slow pace, one that is only 65 percent of your maximum heart rate, your body will adapt and profit from the exercise. You may just be walking and it may not seem like much to you or your friends, but at night as you sleep, your body will say, "Boy, she doesn't exercise very hard, but she sure does a lot of it. I better adapt to this."

▶ Exercise as often as possible.

Lots of books claim that we need to exercise for a half hour three times a week. In this book, I tell beginners to exercise six times a week for twelve minutes. But all of these are just more cumbersome rules. In the end, the rule should be to get out there and exercise as much as you possibly can. We like to see people do lots and lots of exercise.

For example, if I were really fat and terribly out of condition, I would probably exercise five times a day. If you are fifty pounds overweight, find time to exercise morning, noon, and night. You could buy a mini-trampoline and bounce on it in the morning when you first wake up to warm up your body. Don't worry about how hard, how high, how often, how this, or how that. Just bounce on the thing and have fun for about twelve minutes without thinking about it too much. If you look at my three rules above you will realize that you are using your big muscles and you're not getting out of breath.

If you are a working person, see if you can find a place to put a stationary bicycle to use during your break. Once, twice, or even three times a day, get on that bicycle even if you have to eat lunch while you're on it. Or take a walk at lunch while you eat. Decide that for the next three months you won't sit down while you eat. Some worrywart might tell you that you shouldn't eat while you are exercising. Well, you shouldn't if you're doing hard competitive exercise, but going for a fast walk and eating a sandwich is not going to bother your stomach or your muscles. You'll probably eat more slowly and eat less and, in the end, be better off.

In the afternoon get back on the bike for another fifteen minutes, and in the evening perhaps take another walk. Try to do four or five short exercises throughout the day. It amazes me how many rules there are about how often a person should exercise. Just remember — the fatter you are, the more often you should exercise.

If you really want to know what to do, find a twelve-year-old boy and do whatever he does. When he rolls on the floor, you roll on the floor. If he goes for a bicycle ride, you go for a bicycle ride. If you keep up his pace, it won't be long before you are pretty darn fit. Right now that might be too much for you, but you get the idea: do a lot.

▶ Don't even think about distance.

I get a lot of phone calls and letters from people wanting to know how far to jog or bicycle or whatever. They have missed the whole point. It doesn't matter how far you go. What matters is, how many minutes a day do you spend trying to change your body into a fit body? Exercise for time, not distance.

When you exercise for time only, you have two advantages. First, you don't need to find a measured course or track. All you need is a wristwatch. You can go anywhere. Second, you aren't tempted to exercise too hard. There is no final destination you are trying to reach. If you decide to run or cycle faster, it won't make any difference. The time won't go any faster. If you are shooting for a certain distance, you'll try to go faster to get it over with. But you can't hurry up time.

Somebody once remarked that we ought to match exercise minutes with the number of minutes we eat. Just think how many minutes a day you spend shoving food into your mouth. If you were to match even half of those minutes doing exercise, you would probably be fitter than a fox. Ask yourself, "Am I putting in enough time each day to expect my body to change in a positive way?"

▶ Cold weather is not an excuse.

I was lecturing about exercise once in Fargo, North Dakota. Someone said, "Mr. Bailey, do you realize how cold it gets here in the winter? How are we going to go outside and run? Won't it hurt our lungs?" Well, at first I just stopped, because I don't live in a place that gets that cold. Then I thought about it, and my answer was, "How come you went skiing in Colorado last week?" Isn't it funny how we go out to ski or play in the snow without thinking anything about it? We don't come in saying, "That was bad for my lungs." We simply say, "I went out and played in the cold." But the minute someone asks us to run in the cold, we think of objections. That's a joke. Don't use cold weather as an excuse.

▶ Rain is not an excuse either.

I live in Portland, Oregon, and let me tell you, it rains so much here people have webs between their toes. Yet more people run in Portland than in practically any other city in the country. Running in the rain is fun. Go out and get wet and come back and jump in the shower. It's a wonderful experience.

Some of you don't exercise in bad weather because you're afraid you'll fall on the slippery roads, or you'll catch a cold, or your hair will get ruined. Fine. Put an aerobic exercise videotape in your VCR, or get on your stationary bicycle, or go to the gym. No excuses.

▶ Find a sport or make one.

People who make a sport out of their exercise have a real advantage. For example, let's compare using an indoor stationary bicycle and riding a bike outdoors. In theory, they should be the same. It doesn't seem there would be much difference between peddling a stationary bike for fifteen minutes or a road bike for fifteen minutes. But! If you compare 100 people who use outdoor bicycles with 100 who use stationary bicycles, you will find that the outdoor bicycle people are much fitter, stay fitter, and usually are a lot happier.

Why is this? There are many reasons, but the most obvious one is that nobody gets on an outdoor bike for only fifteen minutes. Once you get on the bike, the inclination is to go much farther than you can go in that time. You just keep going and going because it's half exercise and half fun. Another reason outdoor bicyclists are fitter is that outdoor bicycling is associated with friends. You do lots of outings not because you need the exercise but because you like to do things with friends. You don't hear indoor bicycling enthusiasts say to each other, "Let's take our stationary bicycles to the park on Sunday for a picnic."

In addition, there are some very subtle advantages. For instance, when I'm bicycling outdoors, balancing, negotiating turns, and making sudden stops all involve muscles that I don't use on a stationary bicycle. When we bike outdoors, we use the muscles differently and deeper. We use a greater percentage of any given muscle than if we did the same exercise on a bicycle that doesn't threaten to tip over at any moment.

▶ After three months, try a wind sprint.

Don't do wind sprints — or anything fast — during the initial two to four months. At first I just want you to do your walk or your bike ride slow and easy. It should even be a little bit boring in the beginning. After two or three months you may reach a plateau of no further improvement. At that point you might try wind sprints. Read Chapter 16 before you try them. Pick one day out of the week and do one or possibly two wind sprints. Wait a whole week before you do it again to make sure that you don't overdo it.

▶ Forget about calories.

People ask me all the time about calories. They say they've read all my books and heard all my lectures, but they want to know what to eat before they exercise to burn the most calories. Or sometimes they ask, "Does bicycling use up more calories than running? Does running burn off more calories than swimming?" Stop thinking about calories during the exercise. The reason we exercise is to change our body's chemistry, not to burn a lot of calories.

▶ Don't diet.

Most people think of dieting as deprivation. It seems that in America all we think about is eating fewer calories and going on "diets." Well, you can take heart, because I never, never want you to diet. In practice, people need to make just one dietary change: eat less fat. If you don't eat fat, you can eat a lot of food without feeling that you are deprived. You won't feel like you're dieting at all because you aren't! Simply make the decision not to allow grease in your food anymore. The simplest way to do that is to stop putting butter, margarine, mayonnaise, or any other pure grease ON TOP of your food.

What a waste it is for people to get on a good exercise program and then put a pat of oily, 100 percent vitamin-free grease on a piece of toast. There is enough fat *in* our foods without putting more fat on top of them. There are many ways to get fat out of your diet, and I've written an entire book about it. However, to get started, you don't need to read any more books or go to any more seminars. To start getting fit and getting rid of your body fat, do the exercises I have described and avoid fat in your diet any way you can.

▶ Eat often.

What is the opposite of eating often? Skipping meals or fasting, right? Out-of-shape people who go without food experience drops in blood sugar over and over during the day, and these drops precipitate hunger or depression. If you are out of shape, you have a special need to keep that blood sugar up by eating often. You shouldn't resort to gimmicky diets or skipping meals or fasting. You should eat foods that are low in fat and high in complex carbohydrates. And you should eat often, at least six times a day. By the way, I didn't say you should eat lots of food — just spread it out by eating often.

► **If you have any more questions, ask a fox.**

That statement is a little flip. You probably wonder what I mean
by it. I mean, use common sense. If you think you are not ready
to start an exercise program today because you still have too
many questions, you are wrong. *Start right now.* If you have any
more questions beyond the ones answered in this book, you are
really kidding yourself. Get out and go. For example, don't
worry about the time of day for exercise. Do you ask a fox what
time of day he does his aerobic exercise? Do you ask a twelve-
year-old boy when he bikes or runs? Do you tell your dog to be
sure to do his aerobics at ten o'clock in the morning?

The point is, fit creatures just exercise a lot. They get out and
they go. Don't worry about the time of day. If you are a morning
person, exercise in the morning. If you're an evening person, exercise in the evening. Don't let someone with a Ph.D. tell you that
a certain time of day is better than any other time of day. The
right time is up to you and your personality.

Older people sometimes complain that I haven't addressed
their special problems. They are wrong. I do address older people, and I'm addressing you now. It doesn't make any difference
to me if you are thirty or ninety. Get out and do some exercise,
remembering that when you are older, tissues take longer to repair. Obey all the rules in this book, including the rule that you
should go more slowly than younger people. Take it easy, stretch
a little more. Just be careful. For heaven's sake, if you are seventy
years old, you are supposed to be smart by now. Apply those
brains to everything in this book: slow down and use more common sense than a young kid would.

Pregnant women make up objections. They say, "Well, I'm
pregnant and I guess I shouldn't do my running, or bicycling, or
work out at the club anymore." That's pretty silly. After all, a
pregnant fox doesn't stop running. Obviously, if you are pregnant, just take it easy, that's all. Do all the things you would normally do, but just go a little slower.

Many people ask about meals. "Should I exercise before a

meal or after a meal?" Again, I think that is splitting hairs. Some people can eat and exercise and feel fine. Other people eat, exercise, and throw up. If you are one of those, don't eat before you exercise. Don't ask silly questions. Just get out and exercise.

▶ Repeat to yourself while exercising:

"I'M NOT BURNING A LOT OF CALORIES WHILE I'M EXERCISING, BUT MY BODY IS CHANGING INTO A BETTER BUTTERBURNING MACHINE. THE PURPOSE OF MY EXERCISE IS TO CHANGE MY CHEMISTRY."

If you keep repeating that to yourself, you won't fall into the trap of wondering what to eat, how many calories you are burning during the exercise, or whether you are doing it exactly right. It doesn't matter. Get out and do something. Say to yourself, "I need a tune-up and that's why I'm exercising." How your body repairs, changes, and improves *after* the exercise is what matters.

▶ People who skip a day's exercise are useless, lazy, and hopeless.

No! That's not true. We all get lazy and skip a day. In fact, lots of us take a week off now and then. If you don't exercise for a day, don't feel bad about it. Just get back to it when you can, knowing that everyone is like that. In fact, I'll tell you the truth about your author. It is hard for me to write books; I feel drained even though I love it. When I finish this book and send it off to my publisher, I'll probably go for a week without exercising while eating all the wrong foods. I'm not weak, I'm not useless, and I'm not lazy. I'm a normal human being and so are you. If you didn't let that outrageous "lazy and hopeless" statement stop you, you are going to make it. You didn't quit. You kept right on reading the small print down to here, and you'll keep on exercising through the setbacks. Don't be too rigid about the rules, and don't worry if you miss a day now and then.

18

Changing the Shape of Your Muscles

I REMEMBER CAROL, a sad example of overdependence on the bathroom scales. When she started our program, she weighed 127 pounds and was 26 percent fat. After six months of aerobic exercise, Carol had dropped to 23 percent fat. She had lost two inches off her waist, two and a half inches off her hips, and one inch off each thigh. She now wore a size ten instead of a size twelve. She looked better and felt better. But when we weighed her on the scale, she had gained six pounds. Obviously, because of the change in measurements, the six-pound increase meant an increase in muscle mass, which weighs more but takes up less space than fat. But all Carol could see was that she had gained weight. "This is stupid," she said and quit the program. That's what I call shallow thinking.

Most people expect a dramatic weight loss when they embark on an exercise program. Well, I hate to disappoint you, but unless you're quite a lot overfat, there will be little if any reduction in your total weight. In fact, you may *gain* weight. Muscle is much heavier than fat. As the fat is exercised away from inside the muscle, total muscle mass will increase, and it's likely you'll gain two to three pounds, assuming that you were not grossly overweight when you started.

What does change is your shape. Alan was a most dramatic example. Alan didn't think he was overweight, but he had the typical middle-aged pot belly. He started an aerobics exercise program and in six months his waist went from thirty-eight inches to thirty-two inches — *and he didn't lose one pound!* Once a woman sent me a bill for $175 as a joke. This is what it cost her to start a new wardrobe when she dropped from a size twelve to a size eight — *while gaining six pounds.*

Let's look at what happens to muscle when it isn't exercised. All of us start with muscles that are long and lean with very little fat. As we become older and more sedentary, fat slowly invades the muscle. The shape of the muscle itself changes, becoming shorter and rounder. The muscle eventually becomes so saturated with fat that it can't hold any more, and then the fat begins to accumulate outside the muscle, under the skin. When you diet, you lose fat from under the skin. Your diet has little effect on the fat inside the muscle and nothing happens to the muscle shape. It's still short and round. But you can exercise the intramuscular fat away and change the muscle back to its original long, lean shape. Men lose the roll around the middle, and women regain the waist they had in their youth.

It's the fat under the skin that one can see, pinch, and weigh. Obviously, loss of subcutaneous fat will result in change of body size. But usually the person's shape merely seems to be a smaller version of what it was before the loss. You go from a big pear shape to a little pear shape. It's muscles that give your body shape. The definition and firmness are due to exercised muscles, not to loss of subcutaneous fat. As you exercise, keep saying to yourself, "My muscles are getting lean and slinky."

19

Should I Exercise
When I Feel Ill?

EXERCISE PUTS STRESS on muscle tissues, and we expect those tissues to take the abuse and then recover by the time we exercise again. In fact, we hope they will repair so well that they will actually be better than they were at the beginning. In a sense, you are damaging your tissues, hoping that they will respond by getting stronger. You expect not only to repair the tissue protein that you damaged but also to build some new protein. Rebuilding requires protein biosynthesis, which in turn requires that your biochemistry be in good shape and that you eat some protein to provide the building blocks for biosynthesis.

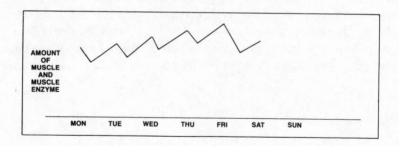

The graph above illustrates the way muscle and muscle enzymes can increase when a person exercises properly on a day-by-day basis. Notice that the amount of muscle and muscle enzyme decreases in the first few hours after exercise. This decrease can be measured by an increase in nitrogen, an essential component of protein, in the urine over the four hours following the exercise. This is followed by a period of very little nitrogen in the urine as the damaged tissues absorb all the protein they can get for biosynthesis. If all conditions are perfect, the person will synthesize more muscle protein than he lost. Over several days, there should be a gradual net increase of body protein. Unfortunately, conditions are *not* always perfect. For example, the person whose muscle changes are shown in the graph exercised too long and strenuously on Friday, and he was unable to resynthesize all that he lost by the time of his Saturday exercise. The result is a net loss over this twenty-four-hour period. He might be able to counteract this effect by allowing more time for the repair phase. You can see that you could have a net loss instead of a net improvement if you overexercised every day.

The body needs energy for an exercise program. If calories are limited, the protein in the diet will be converted to glucose and fat for energy, so the protein won't be available for biosynthesis. The energy demand will always take precedence over protein biosynthesis. It's difficult to pinpoint the minimum calorie level at which protein biosynthesis can take place. I would suggest, however, that men of average size should eat no less than 1500 calories, and women of average size should eat no less than 1200 calories. If you are a woman currently existing on 1000 calories, I urge you not to decrease your intake as you begin an exercise program. In fact, you may well have to increase it a bit. Superfat people in the four-hundred-pound class must *limit* calories to lose fat, but they must *have* calories in order to spare protein. This may be part of the reason that these people have such a hard time losing weight. It may be that their problem is irreversible, but there is no proof as yet.

In general, the older you are, the more slowly your tissues repair, in the same way that cuts and bruises last longer as we get older. This means that the destruction of tissues by hard exercise might not repair completely in twenty-four hours. It's quite possible to have a net loss if you exercise the same muscles too often or too hard. And with age, that possibility increases. Some people in their sixties have undertaken serious, well-intentioned exercise programs, only to have a net muscle loss because they exercised too hard or too often. Their tissue repair doesn't keep up with tissue damage.

If you are sick, your tissue-repairing ability may be somewhat decreased. You can decide if exercise is warranted by figuring out whether or not your "illness" will affect the same tissues as your exercise. Take a sore throat for example. If it is the result of shouting at a football game or too much night life in a smoky room, it shouldn't stop you from exercise. But if that sore throat is part of overall aches and pains like the flu, you had better not run. Overall illness, or systemic illness, will retard tissue regeneration no matter what the exercise. By the way, emotional stress

Muscle loss will occur if	Solution
the exercise is too intense.	• Exercise in the proper heart training range (see Chapters 10, 11, and 12).
there is insufficient time for recovery.	• Age 30 or under — wait 24 hours before next exercise period.
	• Age 30–50 — wait 24 hours before next exercise period *and* switch exercises day by day.
	• Age 50 or older — exercise every other day and change exercises day by day.
you have an illness or disease (including emotional problems).	• Lessen the intensity of exercise if you have a local injury or illness.
	• Don't exercise when systemically ill; the body needs the protein to repair sick tissues.
dietary protein is inadequate or imbalanced.	• Eat 60 grams of protein a day.
	• Be sure the diet is balanced; when carbohydrate is low, protein will be used to make glucose instead of to repair tissue.

can also decrease the recuperation powers of all your body systems. It has been shown that the protein you eat during emotional stress is not utilized as well as usual. During such periods there is a distinct increase in protein waste products in the urine.

Remember! All these factors are cumulative. If you are suffering a mild systemic illness, coupled with some emotional problems, and your diet is poor, exercise probably will do you no good. The older you are, the more likely it is that this will be the case.

20

Spot Reducing

SINCE FAT CONCENTRATES in specific areas of the body, most people feel that those areas must be superexercised to get rid of the fat. Women are concerned about fat deposits on their hips and thighs, and men worry about fat around the midsection. So they are suckered into joining health spas that guarantee to remove fat from specific areas. Or they buy all kinds of pulling, punching, and kneading devices to jiggle away the fat.

There are two favorite modes of spot reducing, passive and active. But neither mode works! In fact, no known technique, short of surgery, will remove fat from a particular place on the body.

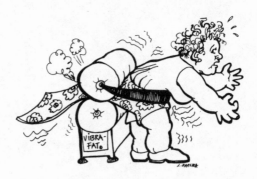

Passive spot reducers include the pulley belts and rollers we used to see in health spas. The theory is that if you beat it long enough, you're bound to break up the fat and disperse it. I can't help thinking that this is the way to prepare Swiss steak. You are not getting rid of the fat — you're tenderizing it. One variation of the rollers, if you can't afford to join a gym, is to simply sit on the floor and bounce up and down on your rear end. Same result — Swiss steak.

The bumpers and rollers, which have pretty much disappeared from health clubs, have been replaced by another kind of fat manipulator — the masseuse. Actually, massage is very beneficial after exercise; it relaxes tense muscles and stimulates the flow of lymph, but some people fool themselves into believing that it actually speeds up fat loss. The only fat loss that occurs from a massage is in the massager, not in the massagee!

Another favorite method of passive spot reducing is tying a heated belt around your midsection. When the belt is plugged in, the heat is supposed to melt away the fat. What do you think is *really* happening? Heat and pressure drive the water out of the tissues in that area. If you remove the belt and quickly tape-measure your waist, you'll be amazed to find you've lost inches! Wait a half hour — the tide will roll back in.

Another popular rip-off is the sweatsuit, a kind of cross between active and passive spot reducing. If you wear the sweatsuit while exercising, believers contend, you'll increase the burning of fat. Let me tell you, *fat boils at 360 degrees!* All sweatsuits really do is increase water loss and decrease your stamina. One of the most dangerous problems in long-distance running is heat prostration, in which the runner cannot get rid of body heat fast enough. When muscles get too hot, the enzymes in the muscles work less efficiently. Enzymes are proteins, delicate chemicals that function best at body temperature and body acidity. Don't try to outsmart your body chemistry by imposing artificial temperatures on it. Wear enough clothes to be comfortable. The best method is to wear layers of clothing and shed the outer garments as you warm up.

It also follows that it is foolish to try to lose weight in saunas or steam baths. These are simply other methods of manipulating body temperature. At best, these practices are unwise if done in excess (you may be destroying those delicate muscle enzymes needed to burn up fat), and they can be downright dangerous if your body is trying to fight off an infection or virus (your temperature will already be elevated). And, of course, any weight loss will be water, not fat.

Now what about active spot reducing? In general, this involves using the muscle that is directly beneath the fat deposit. I'll have to admit I was conned into this myself. I was starting to get a little roll around my midsection, so I did what anyone would do — sit-ups. I did 300 sit-ups a day. I did sit-ups first thing in the morning. I did sit-ups on my coffee break. I'd stick my feet under the tracks and do sit-ups while waiting for the trolley. I'd even hang by my legs from an exercise bar and do sit-ups. Within three months, my stomach muscles were like cast iron . . . but with three inches of marshmallow on top of the muscles.

Women frequently complain about fatty deposits on their upper thighs. So they do leg raises and donkey kicks, or they buy pulleys that loop around the foot and over a door, attached to a weight. They work that poor muscle to death.

In both sit-ups and leg exercises, what you are essentially doing is weight lifting. And when a muscle is exercised by weight lifting, it enlarges (hypertrophies). The end result is a *larger* muscle with that same fat deposit sitting on top of it. The subcutaneous fat on top of a muscle doesn't "belong" to that particular muscle. It belongs to the entire body. And it's only going to get used up if the caloric demand is so great that the fat is needed for fuel. When only one muscle or a relatively small set of muscles is exercised, the caloric demand is small. But when large sets of muscles are exercised, fat is drawn from all parts of the body to meet the energy requirements. It follows that to get rid of fat, you must use your biggest, hungriest (calorie-consuming) muscles. And the largest sets of muscles in the body are in the legs and buttocks — the very muscles used in any aerobic exercise.

The point of all this is, it is impossible to reduce subcutaneous fat from a selected spot on the body. It simply cannot be done!

One can reduce the intramuscular fat by selective exercising of one area, but this will not affect the fat deposited under the skin over those muscles. Subcutaneous fat must be thought of as "belonging to" the whole body. Food in the refrigerator doesn't "belong" to the cook just because the cook is near the refrigerator all the time. Fat under the skin, like food in the refrigerator, is stored for general use. One person, no matter how gluttonous, will take longer to clean out the refrigerator than a whole bunch of hungry but normal eaters. One muscle, no matter how much it is exercised, will take longer to use up the fat on top of it than will a whole bunch of exercised muscles. Get your largest muscles all going at once if you want subcutaneous fat to decrease.

In women subcutaneous fat is usually deposited first on the back of the thigh, then on the outside of the thigh, then on the hips, then on the midriff, and finally in the upper body, particularly under the arms. In most cases, these subcutaneous deposits are removed in reverse order. If you are a woman with fat in those places, and you start a daily bicycle exercise program, the fat will decrease in reverse order from the way it was deposited. Even though bicycling is basically a leg exercise, you will lose fat from your arms first and your legs last.

No matter how many times I tell people to lose fat by systemic (aerobic) exercise, someone inevitably asks how to lose fat from some specific place on the body. Women with fat arms seem to be convinced that arm wiggling, or push-ups, or rubbing, or pounding is necessary to get the fat off their arms. Believe me, if you bicycle or jog, that fat will drain away a lot faster.

That special puckering in women's legs, often called cellulite, is just lots of fat under a slightly different skin texture. It may be driving you crazy, but I warn you not to be suckered into exercises or manipulations of that particular area. Instead of worrying about unsightly fat in one area and trying to change that area, you should get involved in whole-body athletics, particularly aerobic exercises, and trim down all over. Good athletes are never concerned about specific fat deposits.

Part of the confusion about spot reducing probably comes

from the fact that we *can* "spot build." You've probably never heard that term before. In fact, neither have I — I just made it up. Most people call it weight lifting, but isn't "spot building" a fun way to think about it? By changing the shape and size of specific muscles in particular locations, we can alter our appearance dramatically. Even though we can't spot reduce, we *can* spot build.

21

Weight Lifting

Since this book is about fat and getting rid of fat, what, if anything, does weight lifting have to do with helping us get the fat off our bodies? Let me clarify right away that I am talking about heavy weights rather than the one- to three-pound hand-held weights currently popular with aerobic exercise (see page 80).

Years ago I thought weight lifting was a waste of time for fat people. If you look around in nature at creatures that are very low in fat, you'll find that they are always running animals — foxes, deer, antelope, dogs, coyotes. They run and run and are low in body fat. That's aerobic exercise. Very few coyotes do much weight lifting as far as I know. Furthermore, weight lifting burns no fat during the exercise and does not enhance fat burning in the muscles afterward (see Chapter 25). People who *only* weight lift get big muscles that don't burn fat very well. The huge Russian weight lifters are classic examples. They are strong, have lots of muscle — and lots of fat. Weight lifters who are fat are not just eating too much, they also are doing no aerobic exercise with all those muscles.

Although I often compare muscle in a human to the engine in a car, there is a major difference. Cars burn only one fuel. Muscles burn two. Muscles that only have been "weight lifted" owe their strength to their glucose-burning potential. Glucose is the quick-burst fuel that the muscle needs for a major contraction over very short time. It's the same old story, repeated throughout this book: we adapt to whatever we do a lot of. Our muscles adapt to the short but very intense burst of energy required by heavy weight lifting by getting bigger and by getting better at burning glucose, the quick-acting energy fuel. So the weight lifter gets bigger and bigger, stronger and stronger, burns glucose better and better, and his fat waits for the day when those muscles do a long slow aerobic exercise.

Using all these arguments, you might conclude that there is absolutely no point to weight lifting for fat loss. NOT SO! Weight lifting has a significant cross-training effect on control of body fat. I'm referring to the fact that increased physical strength usually makes it easier to perform in sports; weight lifters can run, bicycle, and play basketball with more vigor, burn more calories, and more easily get aerobically fit. If you are already committed to becoming an efficient fat burner via aerobics, the addition of even a little weight lifting will speed up your progress nicely.

Most weight lifters are low in fat and do not fit my description of the fat competitive power lifters. That's because they watch their diets carefully and get into aerobic activities without thinking much about them. They play a little backyard basketball or soccer, both of which lower body fat like crazy, without listing the activity as part of their exercise program. After all, a little basketball is just for fun.

If you can accept that aerobic exercise is primarily fat-lowering and weight lifting is primarily muscle-building, you can better design your exercise time for maximum efficiency. Circuit training attempts to combine the two. There are many permutations, but basically one hurries from one weight-lifting position to another, sometimes using an aerobic machine such as a bike or jump rope in between. Typically the weight used at each station works the muscle to 50 or 60 percent of its potential, and no resting is allowed. Does circuit training work? Yes, it gives some aerobic conditioning and some muscle building; but it is not 100 percent effective at either. Circuit training is great for getting back to exercise after an illness, and it's a great way to "maintain" for a few weeks when you haven't time to do your usual full exercise periods.

Let's keep in mind that weight lifting does not necessarily mean pumping iron in a gym. When you do a sit-up you are lifting a very large weight, the upper part of your body, with a very small muscle, the abdominal muscle. A small muscle lifting a large weight is basically what weight lifting is all about. The same is true if you do squats or push-ups. You're using your own weight as if it were a barbell. You can do push-ups from the floor with your face down, or you can lie on a bench with your face up pushing a barbell up and down, which is called bench pressing. They're almost identical exercises, but one requires expensive equipment and the other requires none. Chin-ups are the classic weight-lifting exercise, requiring practically every muscle in the upper body, from your wrists, arms, and shoulders to the back, and abdominal muscles all the way down to the pelvic girdle. A chin-up is one of the best weight-lifting exercises, yet it requires almost no equipment at all.

The next time you are in a gym, ask yourself as you start each exercise whether the activity is going to have systemic or local effects. Is it basically an aerobic, low-intensity, long-term, easy-breathing exercise? Or is it weight lifting, lasting only minutes, requiring fairly heavy effort and breathing? Weight lifting produces lactic acid burn in muscle and eventual muscle growth. Aerobic exercise produces no lactic acid burn and lowers body fat. Both forms of exercise are excellent.

22

Don't Confuse Work with Exercise

ONE OF MY GOOD FRIENDS, Tim, who is a long-distance runner, recently bought a farm in Oregon. I saw Tim a few months after he moved and asked how he was feeling. "Out of shape," Tim replied. "I've been working so hard that I'm not getting any exercise!" Sounds strange, doesn't it? Tim was up every day at dawn, feeding the animals, milking the cows, plowing the land, piling bales of hay. By the end of the day he was exhausted — yet he didn't feel exercised!

Remember, very few calories are used during any exercise. Be it weight lifting, aerobics, or something else, very few calories are used *during the exercise*. But! Exercise changes us. It increases the metabolic rate, increases the amount of muscle, raises the level of calorie-consuming enzymes inside the muscle, and increases the burning of fats. Sustained exercise at 65–80 percent of the maximum heart rate is very efficient at bringing about these changes. Most jobs involve short bursts of effort, which are inefficient in bringing about these changes. Yes, physical work is a form of exercise, but like weight lifting, it is not effective for fat control.

Women who find themselves in that age-old mother-at-home situation frequently exclaim, "Exercise! I exercise all day long! I chase the kids and mow the lawn and do the dishes, the cooking, and the housekeeping. Why, I never stop exercising!" When I tell them they're not getting any exercise at all, they're ready to slug me.

I realize this might sound confusing, but look at it this way. Suppose the muscle in your arm is capable of lifting sixty pounds. All day long you work that muscle. A housewife may lift twenty pounds of laundry, fifteen pounds of groceries, push that muscle to do ironing, gardening, maybe even to spank her kids. But at no time during the day has she put a *sustained* demand on her body. To the muscle, it's just busywork. She's tired at the end of the day, but the muscle has been worked to only about 50 percent of its capacity. Hence 50 percent of the muscle can give way to fat. The work you do may cause the heart to beat faster, but you rarely sustain the work long enough to get any benefits. Work, in fact, should be put in the same category as weight lifting or sprinting. It is nonaerobic. It is not systemic. It is usually too high or too low in intensity or too short in duration to produce the desired metabolic changes.

Additionally, most kinds of work demand only one set of muscles. Aerobic exercises put a demand on all the muscles of your body, including the heart muscle. You may not think your arms are getting any exercise when you are running, but metabolically they are getting conditioned. Aerobic exercise will get you in condition for work, but work won't get you in condition for exercise.

One of the fattest men I've known was a physician in Sacramento, California. When he was ten, his father died, and from that age on he had to support himself. He did all kinds of strenuous labor from carpentry to hod carrying. Even after he had worked his way through medical school and could afford to sit back and relax, he still kept right on working in every spare moment. When I tested him in the water tank, he came out 55 percent fat! How do you tell this man that all that work doesn't amount to proper exercise?

23

Insensible Exercise

FIT PEOPLE often get involved in exercise without sensing that they're exercising at all. In other words, their fitness allows them to do physical things without being aware of it. We call such unconscious muscular activity "insensible exercise."

Take two housewives who are the same age, height, weight — everything identical except that one is fat and one is fit. The fit woman's "dishwashing rate" will be higher than that of her fat counterpart. When these women go out grocery shopping, the fit one will probably move more quickly and farther and use slightly more calories than the fat one. And so it goes with every other activity.

Time and motion studies have been done to show these differences in activity level in another way. Movies were taken of high school girls in gym class playing volleyball, tennis, and basketball. Later, in a laboratory, the films were slowed down, and each still shot was labeled as to whether the girl in it was active or inactive. During all sports the fat girls had a significantly higher percentage of inactive time than did the fit girls.

Have you ever watched two fat people playing tennis? They have the longest arms! They unconsciously find ways to hit the ball with less running around. They have become so efficient that they hardly move at all. Fat people have adapted to a low activity rate, so they just don't do as much during any given exercise.

When our fat housewife is washing dishes, she is using fewer calories because she has found ways to eliminate unnecessary movement. It's only in the more active sports that this efficiency of motion becomes obvious, and in the very active athletics it becomes a detriment — fat people can't compete.

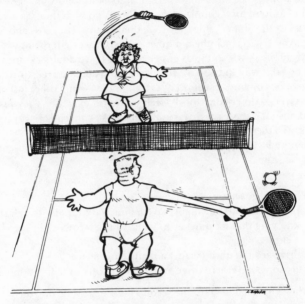

Have you ever watched two fat people playing tennis? They have the longest arms!

Fit people, on the other hand, are inclined toward insensible exercise. They're the ones who shift in their seats during the sermon in church. They're the ones who get up and go to the refrigerator instead of asking the spouse to bring them something. They're the ones who join their kids in a game of Frisbee when the family is on a picnic instead of sitting on a blanket with the Sunday newspaper.

Not only do fat people unconsciously move less, but I've met some who are downright sneaky in finding ways to avoid exer-

How Much Insensible Exercise Do You Do?

If you want to see insensible exercise at its best, follow an eight-year-old kid around for a couple of days. There's no such thing as a "quiet child." At the dinner table they rock their chairs. They fuss and fidget when you try to teach them a quiet game of cards. To them, walking is ridiculous — it's so much easier to run. If we adults skipped and pranced the way kids do all the time, we wouldn't need to read all these books on how to get rid of fat. Children — and other insensible exercisers — don't consciously seek out extra exercise. They just do it because it's the easiest, fastest, and most convenient way to do things. To them it's more fun to be moving than to be still.

Here's a little test you can take to see how you rate on the insensible exercise scale.

1. When you go shopping, do you
   a. park in the first available space and walk rapidly to the store, knowing that it's quicker to walk a little farther than search for a closer space?
   b. drive around until you get a really close space?
   c. get someone else to drive and drop you off at the front door?

2. When you need to go to the second floor in a store, do you
   a. walk up the stairs?
   b. walk up the escalator?
   c. stand on the escalator?

3. On a family picnic, do you relax with a game of
   a. Frisbee?
   b. horseshoes?
   c. gin rummy?

cise. I worked in a San Francisco weight clinic in which all the clients were at least sixty pounds overweight. I remember the day I had Marjorie use the stationary bicycle. I got her adjusted on the bicycle and left her with instructions to pedal five miles. I

4. While waiting for your flight at the airport, do you
   a. walk around?
   b. read a book?
   c. read a book and eat at the snack bar?

5. When getting your luggage after your flight, do you
   a. stand at the far end of the carousel, knowing that it will take less time to carry your luggage the extra distance than to combat the crowds at the head of the carousel?
   b. stand right at the start of the carousel and battle with the other people for position?
   c. hire a redcap?

6. When you drive your car to a service station, do you
   a. fill the tank yourself, clean the windows, and check the fluids?
   b. fill the tank yourself but put the nozzle on automatic so you can wait inside the car?
   c. tell the attendant, "Fill 'er up"?

7. When you hear a record with a beat you really like, do you
   a. automatically get up and start dancing?
   b. stay seated but move your body to the rhythm?
   c. tap your foot?

8. When you're watching television, during the commercials do you
   a. get up quickly to do some little chores?
   b. stay seated but stretch?
   c. ask your spouse to bring you something to eat?

Scoring:
Each *a* answer gets 3 points, each *b* answer 2 points, and each *c* answer 1 point.
22–24 points: You're a high insensible exerciser (or a child!).
12–22 points: You're an average insensible exerciser.
Less than 12 points: You probably have a lot of great hobbies, like stamp collecting and sleeping.

turned to counsel another woman and was surprised when, only a few minutes later, Marjorie appeared at my side. "I'm all done," she said with a satisfied smile. I didn't think Marjorie could have been on the bike for more than three minutes. Besides, she didn't look very sweaty. I didn't want to accuse her of not exercising because it was possible that I had lost track of the time, so I said, "That's great, Marjorie, show me how you did it." What Marjorie had done was loosen the tension device on the bicycle to zero resistance. She then straddled the seat, gave the pedals one good kick, and stuck her feet out as the pedals whizzed by. When they slowed down, she gave them another kick to get them going again. "I pedaled five miles in three minutes at ninety miles an hour!" she said proudly.

In the same weight clinic we used to do an initial test for physical fitness by having the person walk a mile as quickly as possible. We would give the person a stopwatch and a map depicting an exact one-mile route around the streets of San Francisco. We had to find a route that didn't have any shortcuts because people used to cut through alleys, crawl through holes in fences — anything to get out of going the whole distance. It took some people forty-five minutes to walk a mile. They'd have to rest at every telephone pole. I got pretty good at judging how long it would take someone to walk the course, and when Dorothy came into the clinic, I figured she would be gone so long that I would have time to go out for lunch. Well, it's a good thing I didn't take that lunch break because Dorothy was back in twelve minutes! She had taken a taxi! Honest! When she got down to the first corner, she decided this was not her style and hailed a cab back to the clinic.

The point is that by exercising at least twelve minutes a day, we alter our insensible exercise for the rest of the day, and this has far-reaching effects. We end up using more calories in a day because we move more without being aware of it. People incorrectly assume that their calorie needs decrease as they get older because their metabolic rate slows. They picture some mysterious chemical change taking place in their bodies. Not so. Their metabolic rate has not gone down — their activity level has. They are moving less.

24

Set Point — What Is It?

MOST ADULTS HAVE NOTICED that even if their body weight fluctuates, they seem to have a "normal" center point; that is, if they overeat they may gain weight, temporarily, but when they return to a more rational diet, they go back to their usual, or set point, weight. Similarly, a starvation diet may cause you to lose weight, but when you go back to normal eating, you quickly regain pounds and return to your original weight. The implication is that the body resists change in either direction.

For many people the set point seems to be much too high. It's as if their bodies just want to be fat. Lots of fat people, even though they are unhappy with their fatness, admit that their weight is quite stable. This leads to the belief that set point is inherited and unchangeable. If your weight is set at a high, obese point, you may mistakenly believe you are doomed to be fat forever.

Many people overlook a well-known fact: that when they were younger their set point was lower. Lots of people in their twenties maintain a low weight despite wide fluctuations in their diet; when they reach their forties, they stabilize at a much higher level. In other words, set point *can* be changed — it's not an inflexible, inherited affliction one must live with forever.

Set point for body weight does change, but in most people it changes in the upward direction only. The million dollar question is — can your set point be lowered again? The answer is an emphatic yes! You *can* turn down your set point and stabilize your body weight at a lower, healthier point. I freely admit it is harder for some to do this than for others. It's true that we inherit body characteristics, and some people's set points may be harder to alter than others'.

But set point *can* be changed. You can adjust the thermostat in your house by simply twisting a knob. Wouldn't it be great if we could find the right knob in our bodies, give it a quick twist, and watch our bodies adjust to a new fat level? For years people have tried to alter their body weight by dieting, but our body's mechanisms resist any deviation from the point the invisible knob is currently resting on.

As with most complicated issues, the solution to the set-point problem involves a good deal of understanding. We must become aware of a number of factors that raise or lower the number of calories our bodies use. If we can clarify those factors, maybe it will lead us to the secret knob that controls set point.

The body does three things with the calories we ingest. It uses some calories for energy and some for heat production, and it stores the rest as fat. Heat production turns down with age because we tend to wear more clothing and to turn up the heat in the house when we feel chilly. The next time you see some children waiting for the school bus on a nippy morning, note how little they are wearing, while you drive by wearing a coat in your heated car. Children have highly tuned thermoregulatory units. If it's cold, they simply crank out more heat — they use more calories. That's part of the reason children seem to have a hollow leg — they are heating your house with all that food you feed them. As they grow up, they hear constant admonitions to move less. You tell them to stop running in the house. The school teacher tells them to sit still in class. The school bus driver urges them to stay in their seats. As they grow up, they slow down and need ever fewer calories for exercise. At the same time the body's natural control of heat production is lost. This decreased need for calories for heat and exercise is subtle, but it contributes greatly to the turning of calories into fat.

As we lose the ability to produce needed heat, we convert increasing numbers of calories into fat. The fat then acts as insulation for the body so that even less heat is produced. A vicious cycle is established. Body fat insulation increases, central heating turns down, and even more body fat is produced.

I think we do ourselves a disservice when we avoid being a little cold. When children go out to catch the school bus on a chilly morning (without the coat their mother wants them to wear), their bodies adapt in a few moments so that they really are *not* cold. A parent standing beside them, however, feels cold and insists that the kids are cold but are too dumb to admit it.

Thermoregulation is also important when we get too hot. Runners build up a lot of excess heat during a long run, and if the day is hot and humid, they have trouble getting rid of it. During the Peach Tree Run in Atlanta several years ago, more women dropped out with serious heat prostration than did men. It was assumed that women's bodies cooled down less readily than men's. But subsequent laboratory testing of runners has shown that the ability to get rid of heat is related to fitness and body fat level rather than to maleness and femaleness. The women were having more trouble because they were fatter and less fit. Women entering competition today are fitter and have fewer problems getting rid of excess heat.

The point of all this is that we can change the body's ability to create heat and its ability to cool off. Both of these functions are related more directly to our state of fitness than to inherited characteristics.

Heat production is just one of the mechanisms that make up set point. Let's look at another: muscle.

Muscle is unique in its ability to produce sudden bursts of energy. All cells require energy, but cells other than muscle undergo relatively small changes in their energy requirement. For example, brain cells use only twice as many calories during intense thinking as during sleep. On the other hand, when muscle cells go from a resting condition to a sudden burst of energy, their energy demand may increase by fiftyfold in a split second. Muscle also has special enzymes that enable it to burn up tremendous amounts of calories in short periods. It's the only tissue with enzymes that are specialized for sudden increases in calorie burning. Finally, muscle constitutes a large portion of the body, between 30 and 50 percent.

Now let's put these three important facts together. First, muscle uses many calories because movement is more calorie-demanding than any other body function. Second, muscle uses many calories just because a large percentage of the body is composed of muscle. When we add the third fact, that specialized enzymes existing only in muscle can increase calorie burning by fiftyfold during exercise, then it's clear that if you want to burn calories, you should look to the quantity and quality of your muscle.

Muscle accounts for about 90 percent of metabolism. In other words, if you are eating 1,000 calories a day, approximately 900 of those calories will be burned in your muscles. If you lose muscle mass, you lose metabolizing machinery, and your need for calories diminishes. Because you need fewer calories, you get fat on the same number of calories that once *maintained* your weight. Loss of muscle mass doesn't mean you appear smaller. Your bicep may have the same circumference that it had when you were stronger, but now it lacks muscle "tone." Its protein content has decreased and its fat content has increased. Are your muscles soft?

Although I push aerobic exercise because it favorably changes muscle in all three of the ways discussed above, even anaerobic exercise can turn up the set point. It doesn't change the fat-burning enzymes very much, but it *does* change muscle size. Take weight lifting as an example. Weight lifters believe they are using lots of calories when they work out in the gym. They aren't! They are using calories, of course, but not that many. However, as their muscle mass increases, they need more calories during all the other hours of the day. Weight lifting, then, can affect the set point because increased muscle mass means an increase in the number of calories needed to maintain weight. Additionally, weight lifting improves the heat-regulating mechanisms discussed above, thus altering set point from another angle.

People whose set points seem to be too high exhibit yet another metabolic quirk. They handle sugar differently. The ingestion of sugar causes glucose (blood sugar) to rise, and this in turn causes the pancreas to secrete insulin into the blood. The insulin reaches every part of the body and (except in the brain) causes cells to open and admit the glucose, which allows the level of blood sugar to drop again. Muscle cells are supposed to absorb the majority of that glucose. But muscles that have been allowed to get out of shape resist the action of insulin (this is called insulin insensitivity) and hence resist the entry of glucose. The result is that in unfit people, blood sugar is elevated for a longer time after eating. When the glucose is rejected by unfit muscle cells, it is "driven" into fat cells. There it is converted to glycerol, which is then used to produce triglyceride, the body's form of stored fat. Because soft muscles reject glucose, a fat person stores glucose as fat, whereas a fit person stores it as glycogen.

I hope that the set point concept is taking on a whole new meaning for you. It isn't a single weight-controlling mechanism but a combination of many mechanisms.

Hunger control is another factor affecting set point. When fit people engage in exercise, the pH of their blood changes and directly decreases hunger. These blood changes also release endorphins in the brain, which elevate mood and *indirectly* modify hunger by affecting attitude. After all, many of us overeat or eat fattening foods when we are depressed or frustrated. The release of tension and anxiety through exercise helps promote healthy eating. Typically, people with a high set point (a high fat level that stubbornly resists change) are less disciplined about their diets, and they think about food all the time. Fit creatures (including wild animals) eat what they *need*, while fat creatures eat what they *want*.

People with a high set point also have different fat cells. I am not referring to the number of fat cells — that excuse for obesity is no longer tenable. I'm talking about the enzymes in fat cells that convert food into stored fat. These enzymes are especially active in people with a high set point. To fat people this sounds like another doomsday remark. Luckily, this mechanism is also changeable because fat-storing enzymes decrease with exercise.

Your set point can be changed! In case you haven't figured it out by now, I'm telling you exactly where the magical knob of set point is hidden. *Exercise* is the control knob. Exercise lowers set point; lack of exercise raises it. Look at the list of mechanisms below. Exercise changes every one of them. Now you can see why I say diets don't work. Diets may get rid of fat, but they can't turn down the control knob.

What Affects Set Point?

1. Heat production
2. Muscle mass
3. Blood sugar/insulin
4. Hunger control
5. Mood
6. Fat-cell enzymes

> Exercise resets all of the body mechanisms to lower body fat. It is the ultimate control knob of set point.

25

Why Don't Fat People Metabolize Fat?

THE MAIN FUNCTION of fat is to be used by muscle for energy. Almost all diets prey on the misconception that it is hard to burn fat. The fact is that when you are not exercising, 70 percent of the energy needs of muscle are met by fat and only 30 percent by glucose. It's *not* hard to burn fat; we burn it all the time. The sad thing is that fat people burn fat less well than fit people, and this problem is intensified during exercise.

The relationship between fat and glucose burning might best be explained by an analogy. Imagine building a fire in your fireplace. If you put in a big log and light a match to it, what happens? Nothing! The match just goes out. So you put some twigs of kindling wood under the log and light the kindling, which easily ignites. Well, glucose is like kindling; it is easy to burn. Fat, on the other hand, is like a log; it is hard to get started and won't burn well unless some kindling is added once in a while. But it burns for a long time, giving off lots of heat.

Fat, like a big log, contains lots of calories. To keep fat burning properly, you need a little glucose to act as kindling.

Glucose is good for quick energy but, like kindling wood, it doesn't last, so its total calorie value is limited. We use glucose exclusively for energy during a sprint. There just isn't time to get those fat logs burning.

Short-distance runners are glucose burners. Long-distance runners are fat burners.

The enzymes in muscle that burn glucose are quite different from those that burn fat. For some reason, the fat-burning enzymes seem to be particularly fragile. As a person gets out of shape (and fat), the ability to utilize fat for energy decreases rapidly, leaving the glucose-burning enzymes to carry on. One of the characteristics of being out of shape, then, is that your body uses glucose and resists using fat. Hence, the more fat you have, the less fat you burn.

Let's see what happens when a fat person exercises heavily, as shown in the diagram. Keep in mind that for a very fat, out-of-shape person, walking to the refrigerator may be heavy exercise. During heavy exercise, the fat person's muscle burns mostly glucose, since fat-burning enzymes are lacking. This brings down the level of glucose, producing temporary hypoglycemia. Exercise stimulates hunger in a fat person, whereas athletes experience a *decrease* in hunger after exercise. The fat person's hunger may well be due to low blood sugar, although this has not been proven. In any case, he eats, usually including some carbohydrate. The carbohydrate becomes blood glucose, which rises ab-

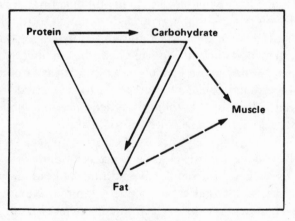

Energy Pathways

normally high because of his insulin insensitivity (see Chapter 24). The high blood sugar, having trouble entering the muscle, enters fat cells instead, where it is converted into fat.

In other words, the fat person who exercises heavily is unable to burn the fat he is trying to get rid of and then makes more fat right after the exercise. He could try to circumvent this by not eating any carbohydrate after exercise, but this would not alleviate the blood sugar problem. The liver would then convert protein into glucose, so he would lose more muscle. And, horror of horrors, he may even lose more of the enzyme proteins — the very proteins he needs to encourage the burning of fat.

The proper way for the fat person to counteract this vicious cycle is as follows. First, exercise very mildly over long periods, because mild exercise allows for the burning of a higher percent-

When Fat People Exercise Too Hard:

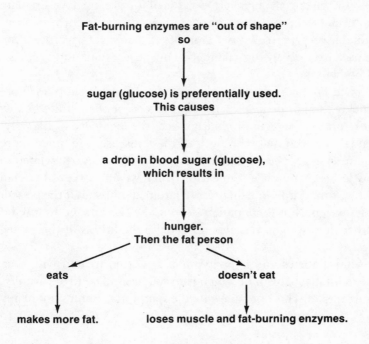

Fat-burning enzymes are "out of shape"
so

sugar (glucose) is preferentially used.
This causes

a drop in blood sugar (glucose),
which results in

hunger.
Then the fat person

eats

makes more fat.

doesn't eat

loses muscle and fat-burning enzymes.

age of fat. Second, eat some carbohydrate, but of the complex type (Chapter 28), which enters the bloodstream slowly. Third, eat this carbohydrate in small quantities six or more times a day.

"Mild" exercise, being a relative term, is best defined as exercise at the lower end of your training zone, about 65–70 percent of your maximum heart rate. It makes no sense to try to burn off fat with bursts of exercise, because you are burning pure glucose. Long, slow exercise gives your muscles time to burn off fat and minimal glucose.

In seasoned athletes, particularly those who do aerobic sports such as running and cycling, the cycle is just the opposite, and it is not vicious. They resist making fat and at the same time burn fat readily. During exercise, the athlete is able to rely on stored fat for calories, thereby saving precious glucose. As mentioned, the exercise does not induce hunger, but if the athlete does eat some carbohydrate, blood glucose will rise more moderately because much of it quickly enters the muscle cells to restore muscle glucose (glycogen). Furthermore, his blood glucose levels remain more uniform, and this eliminates the need for conversion of valuable protein to glucose. Thus the athlete's dietary protein can be used exclusively for its intended purpose, repair and synthesis of body tissue.

Since fat people use up their limited glucose supplies more quickly than fit people, their blood glucose levels tend to be low more often. This will obviously affect the incidence of hypoglycemia and even diabetes. Both of these diseases are much more common in fat people, and it is probable that they are related to low levels of muscle enzyme rather than weight. Every physician knows that borderline diabetes in adults diminishes if the patient loses weight, but these patients should be encouraged to lose fat rather than weight and also to increase the fitness of their muscles.

Mild diabetes and hypoglycemia are often treated with diet, the main mechanism of which is to reduce and control carbohydrate intake. This does alleviate the symptoms, but it's not in any way a cure. If you stop eating carbohydrate because your body can't handle carbohydrate, it's similar to treating a broken leg by saying "don't walk on it." I don't claim for a minute that exercise will cure all blood sugar problems, but there is good evidence that training your muscles to burn fats readily can decrease rapid plunges in blood glucose.

The sad thing about extremely obese people, who often claim they would do absolutely anything to lose weight, is that they refuse to do the one thing that will do them some good. They refuse real exercise, possibly because they associate exercise with sweat and exhaustion. But you see now that the fatter and more out of shape one is, the slower the exercise should be. They must avoid intense exercise like the plague because it will only burn off sugar. For very fat people, a mild exercise such as walking quickly may even be excessive. Their fat-burning enzymes are so low that even the slightest effort shuts off fat consumption. If I were extremely fat, I would give up job, housework, whatever, and I would walk three to four hours per day. I would never give myself a chance to rest, but I would be supercareful not to exceed 80 percent of my maximum heart rate.

26

Is There Anything Good about Fat?

YOU BET there is! For creatures that have to move about the earth for food and sustenance, fat is the greatest thing ever invented. You see, all living things, even plants, have to store a certain amount of food for the times when they can't find or make food. So they store calories either as carbohydrate or as fat. But carbohydrate is a very bulky, heavy form of calories, too cumbersome for mobile creatures. Plants, which don't need to move, store only carbohydrate, while animals store most of their calories in the form of fat.

Most people know that fat contains about twice as many calories per pound as carbohydrate; but there is another, more important reason for animals that move to store energy in the form of fat. When carbohydrate is stored in cells in the body, it is stored as glycogen. Glycogen can occupy only about 15 percent of the space inside a cell. The rest of the space must be left to other functions, most of which require a watery medium. Fat cells, on the other hand, can contain 85 percent fat, leaving only 15 percent of the space for the cell's water-based life functions. This means not only that fat is twice as caloric as carbohydrate but that much more of it can be packed into a small space.

The result is that body fat, being 85 percent pure fat, and

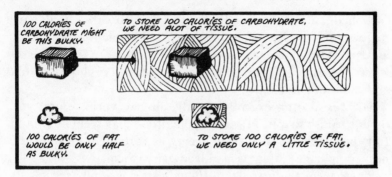

highly caloric, contains about 3500 calories per pound. Contrast this with the liver, which stores carbohydrate as glycogen at only 250 calories per pound. I once calculated that if I were not going to eat for three weeks and I wanted to start out with enough stored calories to last for the whole period, I could use either 9 pounds of fat around my middle or the same number of calories as the glycogen in a 126-pound liver (presumably with a wheelbarrow).

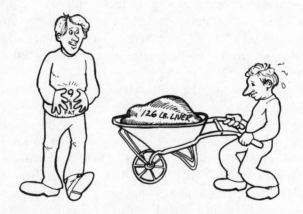

Obviously, a mobile creature is far better off with this marvelous invention called fat. Plants store almost all of their energy as carbohydrate, which is no disadvantage because they don't have to go anywhere. The one exception to this is plant seeds, which are carried by wind, water, or animals to become new plants elsewhere. Seeds contain much fat: hence safflower oil, peanut oil, and sunflower seed oil.

There is also an exception in the animal world. Clams and other shellfish that lie in wait for their food may seem fat, but in fact they are not. They store energy as carbohydrate since the neat compactness of fat is no advantage to them.

Plants were the first living things. After a while, the plants started crawling around on land and we called them animals. This means that carbohydrate was first in evolution, fat appearing only when animals appeared. Hence, fat has a higher evolutionary status. If you are fat, you may derive some consolation by telling your friends that you are unusually high on the evolutionary scale.

Since fat is such a neat bundle of calories, higher animals have evolved many ways of making it. The body can make fat out of protein; the body can make fat out of carbohydrate; and the body can make fat out of fats in the diet — plant seeds or dairy products or meats. In other words, almost everything you eat, if it can be digested at all, can be converted to fat. That's where the problem comes from. And fat people are particularly efficient at converting food to fat.

You must realize that the ability to store food in any form is a great advantage to a living creature. It is like having money in the bank, because it increases your options in life. You should consider stored fat as a safety mechanism. In earlier times, people were, like other animals, occasionally forced to endure short famines. In those times, they could, like the camel, live off their humps. Humans, being a high evolutionary species, have evolved many biochemical routes or pathways for the synthesis of fat and have evolved complex biochemical routes to circumvent the use of that fat and hence to save it.

It has been postulated that one of the reasons fatness is a problem today is that we have inherited the ability to deposit fat very easily. The theory is that our caveman ancestors often had to go days between meals. Those who survived were probably the ones whose bodies were able to adapt to the harsh conditions. And one way of adapting was to carry a little extra fat that the body could live on. Naturally, these primitive people didn't look fat. They were much too active. But they passed on the ability to store extra fat. The body you have today is still watching out for that possible famine and carefully tucking away a few calories out of every meal as fat.

The point of this chapter is to emphasize that your body visualizes fat as a physiological safety mechanism. It reacts to physiological stresses by depositing more fat and using less stored fat. While research has not shown that *every* stress induces this response, many stresses are known to do so. It seems prudent to avoid bizarre weight-loss schemes because the body reacts by increasing fat storage even though you may be losing weight.

There is, for example, good evidence that the popular high-protein/low-carbohydrate diets actually increase the percentage of your diet that is made into fat while you are losing weight. After several months on such diets, even if you have lost thirty pounds, your body has changed so that you have a fat person's chemistry. Your tendency to get fat is greater than when you started!

People who are eager to lose weight sometimes want instant results, but rapid weight loss by any method only augments the tendency to develop a fat person's chemistry. Fasting is another stress that has been shown to make you fatter while you think you are getting thinner (see Chapter 30). Remember, fat is actually very good stuff. Your body will react to radical behavior by attempting to make more fat, even if you are losing weight.

27

The Muscle-*Wasting* Effects of High-Protein Diets

PEOPLE KNOW that fat is especially concentrated in calories, so if they are trying to lose weight, they avoid fat. And there is a common misconception that carbohydrate is fattening, so they also begin to avoid carbohydrates. That leaves protein. In America, everybody eulogizes protein. It started with the reports about protein starvation in India and Africa. Then our coaches and athletes got wind of the idea that muscle is made from protein — and the rush was on. Now proteins are associated with health, life, all kinds of good things. Even hair sprays advertise their protein content. Hot dogs are criticized for being low in protein. Weight lifters pour protein powder into their eggnogs and add it to their ham sandwiches.

Naturally, the most popular weight-loss diets push high protein and low carbohydrate and fat. But how do you get a high-protein diet? By eating lots of meat, right? Well, in case you haven't noticed, meats, particularly in America, are very high in fat. In fact, it's the fat content that makes our meats taste so good. The more expensive the steak, the more intramuscular fat it has. That means that a high-protein diet is really a high-protein *and* high-fat diet. In fact, the most popular low-carbohydrate diets contain so much meat, and therefore so much fat, that they are higher in calories per mouthful than a high-carbohydrate diet.

People do lose weight on high-meat/low-carbohydrate diets, however. One reason is that fat in food slows down digestion quite a bit, so you feel satisfied with less food. Another reason for their seeming effectiveness is that high protein consumption tends to cause loss of body water. If you lose ten pounds on a high-protein diet, two or three of those pounds may be water of dehydration. Later your body reabsorbs the water and you re-gain that portion of your weight loss, making the diet much less effective than it seemed.

But this isn't the major criticism of high-protein, high-fat/low-carbohydrate diets. The big danger is that they are conducive to muscle loss and to degeneration of muscle tone and efficiency.

Since fat, carbohydrate, and protein are the only sources of calories in the diet, the various weight-loss diets consist of end-less manipulations of these three kinds of food. What few people realize is the wondrous way the liver manipulates these food-stuffs for you. Once digested and in the bloodstream, they are

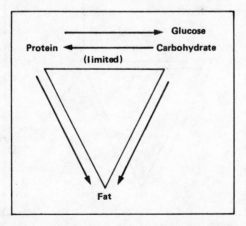

Possible Interconversions of Foodstuffs in the Liver

carried to the liver, which readily converts one form to another, as shown in the diagram. Your body needs all three — fat, protein, and carbohydrate — of course, and the liver is so sensitive to those needs that it starts interconverting very quickly if you eat a particularly unbalanced meal. Your liver seems to be saying, "Go ahead, dummy, eat that ridiculously unbalanced meal; I'll straighten it out." You may have some smart new idea that your body needs less of this and more of that, but believe me, your liver is a lot smarter than you are.

Notice in the diagram on page 128 that although many interconversions are possible, there are no arrows leading away from fat. Fat is never converted into protein or carbohydrate. When I drew the triangle I was in a pessimistic mood, so I put fat at the bottom to indicate that an excess of anything in the diet always leads in a downhill direction — to fat. And who wants fat in the bottom! The only thing your body can do with fat is burn it in the muscles, as shown in the following diagram.

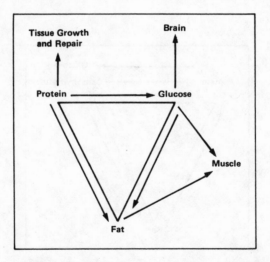

Pathways for the Burning of Fat, Glucose, and Protein

Notice also that protein can be converted into glucose. When people think of glucose, they usually think of muscle, because muscle burns glucose for energy. But muscle can exist without glucose. The essential thing about glucose is its use by the brain. The brain *must* have its glucose! Ask people who suffer from hypoglycemia how they feel when their blood sugar is low. They get woozy, dizzy, and sometimes have blurred vision. When you are not exercising, your brain uses two-thirds of the glucose in your blood. Just think what that means — an organ weighing only one to two pounds is burning up 66 percent of your circulating glucose while your thirty to seventy pounds of muscle scrapes up the rest. In other words, when you are not exercising, one pound of brain burns sixty-six times as much glucose as one pound of muscle. The brain is quite a glucose hog.

Furthermore, although the brain can't function without its glucose, the muscles can! If you exercise too much, your muscles use too much glucose and your brain experiences the symptoms of sugar shortage that I just mentioned. This is one of our built-in safety mechanisms. I'm sure that when the good Lord made us, He knew we would be foolish creatures, the only creatures who think that exercising to the point of exhaustion is play. So if we go too far, we faint from lack of brain food. It's hard to exercise when one is unconscious, so the liver gets a chance to build up the glucose supply by converting protein to glucose.

The point of all this is to emphasize that the conversion of protein to glucose is a powerful body function, one that operates if you endanger the blood glucose supply in any way. For many years it was assumed that the glucose stored in the liver, called glycogen, was the principal source of blood sugar between meals. But now it has been shown that the liver hoards its glycogen. Instead of giving it up for blood sugar, the liver converts protein to glucose.

If you subsist on a bare starvation diet, either voluntarily to lose weight or involuntarily, as in a prison camp, you will convert valuable body protein to blood sugar for your brain. You will lose muscle, the very tissue you need most to burn up the food you eat. If the diet is not only low in calories but also extra low in carbohydrate, you will lose body protein even faster. Typical high-protein/low-carbohydrate diets are usually as low in total calories as a prison camp diet, and they are devastating to body muscle if practiced for any length of time.

It seems odd that a diet that emphasizes protein would cause a loss of body protein, but it does because the total calorie intake is so low. For up to two hours after a meal, your body can use the protein in that meal to make glucose if the carbohydrate in the meal was low (a rather expensive way to get your blood sugar), but after that there isn't any more dietary protein even if you had a high-protein meal. Two and a half hours after a meal, all of the protein in that meal has been used in some manner and is no longer available for the production of glucose. Now how is the brain going to stay alive until you feed it again? The answer is that the body will feed on itself. It will break down its own muscle tissue (protein) and make it into glucose. This process will occur whether you eat a balanced diet or an unbalanced high-protein/low-carbohydrate diet. But the catch is this. The protein you eat should be used to repair tissues that have broken down during the time you weren't eating. Instead, in a high-protein/low-carbohydrate diet, the protein is needed immediately for the production of glucose, and muscle tissue does not get replaced. (In a well-balanced diet, the carbohydrate in the meal is used for glucose production, leaving the protein available for muscle repair.) The net result of a high-protein/low-carbohydrate diet is that the muscles break down and are not repaired, with a consequent loss of lean body mass. As I said earlier, it's possible to lose as much as one pound of muscle for every pound of fat lost on one of these diets.

Most experts agree that approximately sixty grams, or two ounces, of protein a day is enough to meet the needs of the body *and* supply the additional protein needed just in case the person is lactating or pregnant, has the flu or a broken leg, or is lifting weights. A high-protein diet that contains excess calories, such as the diets used by weight lifters who are trying to *gain* weight, will not cause a loss of muscle.

What happens when you eat too much protein? What happens to amino acids (protein) in excess of the body's requirements? When amino acids aren't needed, they're sent to the liver, where they're deaminated and then converted into FAT. Not only that, the process of deamination can be stressful if your body has to do a lot of it. During deamination, the nitrogen that is released from the amino acids is quickly converted into ammonia. Ammonia is very toxic to the body so it, in turn, is changed into urea. Urea is also toxic to a lesser extent, and to be eliminated from the body, it must be diluted into urine. In a normal, balanced diet in which protein constitutes about 12–13 percent of the total caloric intake, your body can very easily rid itself of urea. But what happens when you suddenly increase the protein intake? You've got to get rid of the urea, and you're going to need enormous amounts of water to dilute it. You may drink a lot more water, but it won't be enough. Inevitably, your body will have to take water from its own tissues to dilute the urea. You've suddenly put a very stressful burden on your kidneys, which are working overtime to get rid of the urea. Oh yes, you're losing weight like crazy, but most of it is water loss. Your body may lose up to twelve pounds in water alone on a high-protein/low-carbohydrate diet, regardless of how much water you drink.

How can you be sure you're getting enough protein in the diet while also getting a good balance of carbohydrate and vitamins? A reasonable rule of thumb is to eat two servings daily of three ounces of a meat product (preferably low-fat meats such as chicken and fish) or, better yet, a meat substitute (split peas, dried beans, lentils). In addition, have two servings (one cup each) of nonfat or low-fat milk or a milk substitute such as yogurt, low-fat cottage cheese, or cheese (one slice is a serving). Balance these high-protein foods with carbohydrate by eating four servings of fruits or vegetables each day and four servings of high-fiber breads and cereals, which are grain products (discussed in Chapter 28). To determine a serving size of fruits/vegetables or of a grain product, picture the food broken up into bite-size pieces. If it would almost fill a cup (three-quarters of a cup), then it's a serving.

While it's important to balance your diet with adequate amounts of protein and carbohydrates, you do not have to worry about getting enough fat. It is almost impossible *not* to get fat in the foods you eat. Even if you decided to eliminate all animal products that are high in fat, you would still get fat in nuts and other seeds, including wheat germ.

28

Why Eat Fiber?

LET'S LOOK AT the variety of carbohydrates found in just one food, such as corn on the cob. As you can see from the diagram below, one kernel of corn contains the full range of carbohydrate complexities. When tables of nutrient content were first derived, corn was determined to be only 2 percent indigestible because hemicellulose and lignin were not yet recognized. In those days

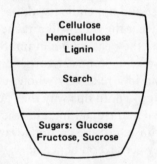

The Complexity of Carbohydrates in Corn

the corn was put into a glass, ground up, and "digested" with acids and alkalies found in the laboratory. After the digestion, 2 percent was left. Recently, however, independent laboratories in England have done a more realistic digestion of corn using enzymes from the human digestive tract. With these methods, 12 percent was left as indigestible, and further research exposed a whole new set of carbohydrates called lignins and hemicellulose. In other words, corn is much less digestible than the nutrition tables had indicated. Most people have noted from personal experience that corn doesn't digest very well.

Corn is a cereal grain, as are rye, wheat, rice, barley, and oats. All of them have similar characteristics, with the fiber carbohydrate forming the outside layers. The outside layers of grain kernels can be cracked off in tiny flakes called bran. Bran is nothing more than the fiber carbohydrate from grain. You would think there was something magical about it the way it was pushed at one time. But bran is only one form of fiber. Furthermore, if you are increasing fiber in your diet by sprinkling bran on other foods, you are not getting the nutrition in the grain kernel underneath the bran.

The studies from Africa showing the advantages of a high-fiber diet do *not* extol the virtues of pure fiber; it's fiber *foods* they are talking about. Africans, protected by their diet from colon cancer, diverticulitis, and appendicitis, do *not* sprinkle bran on their Cheerios. They eat the bran still attached to the rest of the grain kernel; that is, they eat *whole* grain. Some cultures with high-fiber diets eat wheat, some eat corn, some eat rice; but all of them eat the grain in a relatively whole, unrefined condition close to the way it's grown. In this way they get the full gamut of carbohydrates shown in the diagram, plus the vitamins and minerals associated with each of the carbohydrate layers. By eating the whole grain, they get several benefits:

1. The caloric value of the food is decreased by the fiber.
2. Fiber is hard to chew, thus decreasing the tendency to overeat.
3. The fiber gives some protection to the digestive tract.
4. They eat their vitamins *in* their food as nature intended.
5. The simple sugars provide flavor but are delayed in entering the bloodstream.

We are urged to eat more fiber, but nobody ever mentions that *fiber is carbohydrate*. It is odd that while carbohydrate has almost become a dirty word, fiber has become a magic word. Yet they are the same thing. Although there is a great deal of difference between one carbohydrate and another, all of them have certain chemistry in common. For example, all carbohydrates, after intestinal digestion, become the simple carbohydrate called glucose. It's just that some carbohydrates break down in the intestine very quickly, some very slowly, and some (like cellulose) not at all. The complex carbohydrates become blood glucose very slowly, while the simple sugars such as maltose, lactose in milk, and table sugar become blood glucose almost immediately. Complex carbohydrates may even decrease the availability of the sugars in a food.

The people who encourage us to eat fiber are right. We should eat more of that form of carbohydrate. We should decrease the amount of simple carbohydrates because they are, in a sense, predigested and cause our blood glucose levels to fluctuate too quickly. I URGE YOU TO INCREASE YOUR CARBOHYDRATE CONSUMPTION, BUT ONLY BY EATING MORE OF THE COMPLEX VARIETY.

29

How Much Fat Should I Eat?

I CAN ANSWER that question in three words: DON'T EAT FAT! End of chapter. Next question.

Whenever I tell my audiences not to eat fat, someone always worriedly raises his hand and asks, "But shouldn't I eat some fat? Isn't it essential that some fat or oil be included in the diet?" That's true; some fatty acids (for example linoleic acid, linolenic acid, and arachidonic acid) are not synthesized by the body, so they must be obtained from the diet. But if you're eating a four-food-group balanced diet, it's virtually impossible *not* to get these essential fatty acids. Even if I urged you to eat no fat at all, you would inevitably get enough fat in your food. After all, where does corn oil come from? Corn, right? So if you eat corn, you will get corn oil. Similarly, whole wheat bread contains wheat germ, which contains oil. The omega-3 fatty acids in fish have been shown to be of some benefit in the prevention of heart disease. Does that mean we should put fish oil on our food? Of course not! Eat fish! Quit squeezing the oil out of food. Don't put corn oil (margarine) on your food — eat corn! Eat the real thing. Don't eat Wesson oil, eat wessons (whatever the heck they are).

My point then is that even on a very low fat diet, you will probably get the essential fats you need. This is especially true if you are increasing the amounts of whole grains, whole fruits, and vegetables. Such foods supply essential fatty acids and the fat-soluble vitamins A, D, E, and K.

People also get hung up about what *kind* of fat they should eat. Should it be saturated or unsaturated, poly or mono? There's good evidence that saturated fat (the kind that comes from animal products) is more dangerous to the cardiovascular system than unsaturated fats. So, the American Heart Association urges us to eat less saturated fat. However, the American Cancer Society urges us to decrease polyunsaturates because they may contribute free radicals, which are associated with cancer. Both organizations should put less emphasis on which kind of fat to eat and instead urge us to eat less fat and oil of any kind.

It's great to see all the low-fat products that are now available. There are delicious low-fat frozen dinners, no-oil salad dressings that are as thick and creamy as the real thing, nonfat fresh and frozen yogurts. Even animals are being bred and raised to produce leaner cuts of meat. Most magazines today contain several low-fat recipes, and even fast-food chains devote part of their menus to reduced-fat items. It's much easier today to follow my "Don't Eat Fat" rule than it used to be.

Still, for most Americans, approximately 45 percent of the calories we eat are in the form of fat. The American Heart Association used to recommend a 30 percent fat diet and now urges a 20 percent fat diet. Is that hard to do? Not really. A few simple changes such as switching to nonfat milk, never buttering your bread, eating red meats no more than twice a week, and using salad dressing made without oil should do the trick.

When fat people find out how easy it is to start my exercise program, they say, "Oh! I can do that!" Well, making dietary changes should be just as easy. Don't try to make radical changes at first. Just pick one fat food and stop eating it (or eat its low-fat substitute). Tell yourself, "I'll stop eating ice cream and eat nonfat frozen yogurt instead." A month later stop putting butter on your bread and potatoes. Bread tastes great without butter if it's good bread. Moisten your potato with nonfat ranch-style or blue cheese salad dressing. You'll be surprised how great it tastes. There are all kinds of fun and delicious ways to get the fat out of your diet. I've written an entire book on the subject (*The Fit-or-Fat Target Diet*) with chapters on how to shop for, prepare, and eat low-fat foods. Get it and read it!

The chart below gives my recommendations for fat and calorie intake. Unlike the American Heart Association and most diet plans, I do not make the same calorie or fat recommendations for everyone. People, after all, are different. Fit people can afford more calories and more dietary fat. A Category I person does not need to be as restrictive as a Category II person.

If you are fat and/or unfit, your diet should be quite strict, but don't be discouraged. Take it easy! Approach eating in the same way I told you to tackle exercise. Change a little bit at a time. Lots of small dietary changes coupled with lots of small exercise sessions work best.

Recommended Daily Calories and Grams of Fat

| | If your percentage of body fat is | | If you don't know your percentage of body fat* but you | You should eat | | | |
| | Men | Women | | Calories/Day | | Grams of fat/Day | |
				Men	Women	Men	Women
Category 1 (25% fat diet)	15% or less	22% or less	are satisfied with your present weight	2400–2700	1700–2000	No more than 75	No more than 55
Category 2 (20% fat diet)	16–26%	23–35%	want to lose 5–15 lbs.	1800–2200	1400–1700	40–50	30–40
Category 3 (10% fat diet)	27% or more	36% or more	want to lose more than 15 pounds	1400–1800	1000–1400	15–20	10–15

*Caution: Using weight as your criterion is not smart. Have your body fat tested.

30

Fasting

WHEN IT IS DEPRIVED OF FOOD, the body is stressed and tries to lay down extra fat for the emergency. In other words, *fasting encourages the body to become fatter.* A study of rats illustrates this phenomenon. Fifty rats were separated into two groups. Both groups were given exactly the same daily quantity of food. Group A rats ("Nibblers") could eat the food all day long, but Group B rats were allowed only a half-hour to consume all the food ("One Big Mealers"). It took the One Big Mealers a little while to get used to it, but once they realized that no more chow was coming for twenty-three and a half hours, they gobbled up all of their allotment in the half hour. The amount of food was small, and both groups lost about the same amount of weight.

At the end of six weeks, the rats were allowed to return to a normal amount of food, and the One Big Mealers were allowed to be Nibblers again. Both groups gained weight, but the One Big Mealers gained more weight. The researchers analyzed the enzymes in rats that are responsible for the depositing of fat. The Nibblers had no increase in fat-depositing enzymes. In contrast, these enzymes in the One Big Mealers had increased nearly tenfold during the low-calorie diet period. Even though the rats were losing weight because their total caloric intake was low, their bodies seemed to be saying, "The minute more food comes along, I'm ready to lay down extra fat just in case this stress happens to me again!"

In other words, if you *have* to diet, don't make the mistake of fasting or eating just one meal a day (essentially a twenty-three-hour fast). Spread those calories out over the day in five to six small meals. Otherwise you're setting your body up for a heavy fat gain the minute you go off the diet.

This increase in fat-depositing enzymes doesn't last forever. They eventually go back to normal if you stop dieting. But in the rats it took eighteen weeks for the enzymes to go back to normal — three times the amount of time it took to get them out of balance.

Now if you can visualize that fat was originally meant to be a marvelous advantage to mobile creatures and that it represents a magnificent safety device against famine, you can appreciate that the body will attempt to make more of it under most stress circumstances. Temporary fasting is a stress! Even eating only one meal a day is translated by the body as a twenty-three-hour fast, causing a higher percentage of the food you eat to be made into fat. Hence, less food is available for energy and for tissue repair. Likewise, most diets that are high in protein and low in carbohydrate are translated as an emergency situation, causing an increase in the depositing of fat.

31

Contradictory Advice

YOU WILL UNDOUBTEDLY encounter information that seems to contradict what you have read here. Be sure to find out if the advice or research being offered pertains to fat people or to fit people. For example, my cautions regarding exercise, especially not to overexercise, are intended for the 99 percent of the population that is not involved in competitive athletics. The chapter on wind sprints is included for my athlete readers. Wind sprints can be applied in many sports but, illustrated with running, the technique involves running hard for perhaps 150 feet, followed by jogging until you get your breath back. Without ever stopping, you alternately jog and sprint. This technique is well proven to be effective training for competitive athletes. But it doesn't apply to the other 99 percent of us until we are reasonably fit.

The point is that you will hear about many techniques over the years that may well be effective for the trained athlete but are not good for the other 99 percent of the population. Even fasting, which I totally discredited in Chapter 30, may have some benefit for marathon runners. Their bodies handle such stress quite differently. Sugar consumption is still another case in point. Unquestionably, we all eat too much of it; it devastates the teeth and promotes a host of other problems. On the other hand, for seasoned athletes in the midst of competition, a mouthful of sugar is a great help.

Here is another confusing issue. Research studies done by top scientists at Harvard showed that a ten-week exercise program had no effect on obesity. If you read the study, however, you would find that they started with people averaging 450 pounds and 80 percent body fat. Ten weeks of exercise, the researchers claimed, did not diminish the subjects' tendency to get fat. Well, of course not! The subjects may have dropped to 75 percent fat, but they were still very fat people with fat people's chemistry. They were still insulin insensitive and still unable to metabolize fats. For such obese people, exercise reduces only subcutaneous fat and has little effect on musculature. Furthermore, when fat people exercise, it increases their hunger. If these people exercised gently for a much longer time, they *would* be able to change their chemistry.

Even advice on eating before exercise is misunderstood by well-intentioned but mistaken coaches. If you are going into a competitive event, it is bound to be at maximum stress, which is *an*aerobic. Under anaerobic stress, blood flow to the digestive organs is greatly restricted, and digestion can be impeded. So, if you undertake a *hard* run right after breakfast, you may well get sick to your stomach. Kids who go swimming right after a meal may also be more likely to get cramps, since most kids swim with anaerobic bursts. But I am urging GENTLE aerobic exercise! Radical changes in blood flow, digestion, and adrenalin secretion are not typical during aerobic exercise. A sensible meal followed by aerobics is okay for most individuals.

Similarly, advice about warming up and cooling down is sometimes exaggerated. Of course, both are necessary, but they're much less critical for the recreational athlete than for the competitive athlete. Warming up and cooling down by doing a slower version of the activity for five minutes is all the average noncompetitive exerciser usually needs.

Let's assume that 1 percent of the population is extremely athletic and into competition. Let's also assume that about 4 percent of the population is extremely obese, more than a hundred pounds overweight. That leaves 95 percent of the people in the United States in the middle who will not go wrong following the advice in this book. Unfortunately, most of the advice on exercise comes from the competitive 1 percent, so it doesn't apply to the majority of us. Most of the research and advice on overweight comes from work with extremely fat people who abhor exercise, and that doesn't apply to you and me either.

32

Just a Quick Question, Mr. Bailey

IT ALWAYS makes me smile when someone says, "I have just a quick question." His "quick question" usually requires a very involved answer. Every week I receive dozens of letters regarding problems people have with their exercise programs. I would love to answer each of them individually, but I haven't the time or staff to do it. I have included here a bunch of my reader's quick questions and my answers. Perhaps you'll find an answer that applies to your specific problem.

Dear Mr. Bailey,
  I am female, thirty years old, 5' 5", and weigh 135 pounds.
I had a body fat test (water immersion method), which
calculated that I am 16 percent fat. According to your book,
this is low fat for a woman. But 135 pounds seems much
too heavy for my height. I run every day for about an hour
doing eight-minute miles. I eat about 2000 calories a day.
According to the height/weight charts, I should only weigh
about 120 pounds. What should I do to lose 15 pounds?
Eat less? Exercise more?

Sincerely,
Becky M.
Chicago, Illinois

Dear Becky,

I've received many, many letters from women like you who are extraordinarily fit yet worried because they don't have the "ideal" female body. Fortunately, ideas are changing, and we're seeing more and more magazine ads with very feminine women using their well-muscled arms to hold up some new product. These women look beautiful and trim, but with that kind of musculature they certainly aren't the Twiggy-type models of yesteryear.

No! You do not need to lose weight! At 16 percent fat, you're way below the average, which is 32 percent for women. You're even lower than the 22 percent fat I routinely recommend for most women. Women with your fat percentage are often aerobic dance instructors, body builders, gymnasts, or long-distance runners. By the way, since you were tested by the water immersion method, I don't doubt its accuracy. You can sometimes get wrong results with this test if you retain air (gas in the intestinal tract, air in your swimsuit, or incomplete exhalation), but that would give a fat percentage *higher* than your actual percentage. It's almost impossible to get a reading that is *lower* than your actual percentage.

From 16 percent body fat, we calculate:

135 pounds × .16 = 22 pounds of fat
135 pounds − 22 pounds fat = 113 pounds lean body mass

Let's look at these numbers: 22 pounds of fat and 113 pounds of lean. Is 22 fat pounds too much? No, most healthy women (and men, by the way) carry 20 to 25 pounds of fat. Is 113 pounds of lean too much? If you look at the lean body mass chart in Chapter 7, you will see that most women your height have 83 to 99 pounds. With your 113 pounds of LBM, you carry some 14 pounds of bone and/or muscle more than the average woman of your height.

Should you try to lose lean? NO!!! If the extra weight is due to heavier-than-average bones, it would be almost impossible to lose lean unless you cut off a leg. If your large LBM is because you have lots of muscle, you could lose it by going on a very severe, muscle-wasting diet which, in the end, would be the same as cutting off a leg in terms of overall impairment of good health.

Stop worrying about your weight and accept your good luck in inheriting a strong, healthy body. Slaughter all the other women at tennis and be the ideal backpacking companion who carries her share of the load without complaining.

Dear Mr. Bailey,

I am six feet tall and weigh 150 pounds. I eat over 3500 calories a day just to keep my weight up. I don't do much exercise because it makes me lose weight. I recently had a body fat test and they told me I was 24 percent fat. They said that if I wanted to be 15 percent fat, I should weigh 135 pounds! I don't see how they could have recommended such a ridiculously low weight when I look so thin at my present weight.

John A.
Minneapolis, Minnesota

Dear John,

When we test people at our clinic, we routinely tell them what they should weigh in order to be a healthy 15 percent fat (or 22 percent fat for women). From your results we calculate:

150 pounds × .24 = 36 pounds of fat
150 pounds − 36 fat pounds = 114 pounds of lean body mass

From this information, we need to ask two questions. First, how much fat should we add to your 114 pounds of lean in order to make you a 15 percent fat man? In your case, we need to add 21 pounds of fat, because your total weight should be 135 pounds. (For my math-oriented readers, this calculation is done by dividing 114 by .85, the reciprocal of .15.) In other words, a weight of 135 pounds would make you a healthy 15 percent fat. It would also probably make your wife leave you and give your friends the impression that you were ill!

The obvious solution here is to increase your lean so that you can weigh 150 pounds without being too fat. Since the answer to my first question gave an unrealistically low weight, we now need to ask, "How much lean do you need to add in order to be 150 pounds and 15 percent fat?"

$$150 \text{ pounds} \times .15 = 23 \text{ pounds of fat}$$
$$150 \text{ pounds} - 23 \text{ fat pounds} = 127 \text{ pounds of lean}$$

In other words, you need to add 13 pounds of muscle to your present 114-pound frame while losing 13 pounds of fat. You've been eating like crazy trying to maintain your present weight, and all you've been adding is fat. You can't add muscle by just eating a lot. To stimulate muscle growth, you must exercise. All those calories you've been eating can be converted into muscle instead of stored fat if you exercise. Reduce your calorie intake to around 3000 calories a day and start doing about thirty minutes of aerobic exercise every other day. This alone won't change your body much since aerobic exercise doesn't build muscle. But you need to start out this way in order to "wake up" the enzymes in your muscles and get them functioning properly. After about six months, add a body building program on your nonaerobic days. You're a slender man, so you probably won't end up looking like the Hulk. Larger-framed men can easily gain 13 pounds of muscle in a few months, but you should shoot for a 5- or 6-pound gain of lean in a year. (Slender women can usually add 1 to 2 pounds a year.)

By maintaining your present 150-pound weight but slowly changing the fat to lean ratio, you'll be surprised at how much better you look. Your waistline will slim, your shoulders will broaden, there'll be less flab in your arms, and your legs will be firm. Men who weigh 150 pounds and are 15 percent fat look a lot more rugged than men of that weight who are 24 percent fat.

Dear Mr. Bailey,
I've been body fat tested by the water immersion method
and by skin calipers. On one test I was 22 percent fat and on
the other I was 34 percent! Which one is correct?
                                                    Gloria J.
                                                    Twin Falls, Idaho

Dear Gloria,

You didn't specify which test gave you 22 percent and which gave you 34 percent, so I can only tell you some generalized things we look for when we get widely divergent results.

We believe that the water immersion test is usually the more accurate. If your result from the water test was 22 percent, believe it! It's very difficult to do the test incorrectly and get a result that is too low. You nearly always get a number that is too high if the test isn't done right. The number-one culprit is air. People who are frightened of water sometimes don't exhale as completely as they should. People who eat beans the day before or drink carbonated beverages the day of the test have more air in their intestines. Even premenstrual women who complain of feeling "bloated" get higher readings than usual. Air makes you float the same way fat makes you float. If you have any kind of air trapped in your swimsuit, your hair, your lungs, or your intestines, the test figures your increased floatability as excess fat and gives an erroneous result.

We like skin calipers because they are easy to use, but in the hands of an inexperienced operator, the results can be way off. We tend to have more problems with women than with men. In men it's fairly easy to separate fat tissue from muscle tissue, but women's musculature is often less defined. The calipers are supposed to pinch fat only, but the operator may inadvertently get muscle as well, which would yield high results.

Skin calipers measure subcutaneous fat (the fat under the skin). Based on this measurement, they give an *estimate* of total body fat. In most cases, this estimate is fairly accurate, being within 1 or 2 percent of water immersion readings. But sometimes there is a considerable difference. Extremely fit athletes usually get higher skin caliper results because their subcutaneous fat may be average, but their intramuscular fat is extremely low. Swimmers often get high skin caliper readings despite lean muscles because they carry more protective skin fat. In contrast, very thin nonathletic people get lower skin caliper results because their low subcutaneous fat masks the fact that inside they're loaded with intramuscular fat.

Basically, you have to look at your exercise and diet habits. If you exercise frequently and eat a low-fat diet, the 22 percent reading is probably correct. If you don't exercise much and you eat a lot, the 34 percent results are probably more accurate. If you go on a lot of weird diets or if you fast frequently, your lean body mass may be low, in which case the body fat percentage reading appears high even though your total weight may be normal.

In any case, start a regular exercise program and eat sensibly. Hopefully, this reply has helped you decide which of the two tests is more accurate. In six months get another test. The real value of testing yourself is not in the numbers but in whether there is improvement from one test to the next.

Mr. Bailey,
I've been exercising twelve minutes a day for two months and I've seen absolutely no improvement. I'm just as fat as ever. I'll give it one more month and then I'm quitting!
B.T.
Miami, Florida

Dear B.T.,
Your letter doesn't give me much information. If I were able to talk with you, I'd want to know:

1. Have you changed your eating habits? Unfortunately, I may have misled the readers of the first *Fit or Fat?* by implying that twelve minutes of daily exercise was *all* they needed to lose fat.

A lot of people even felt justified in eating more food because they were now exercising. Unless you're a superfit athlete who exercises hours and hours a day, there is no exercise program that can overcome the bad effects of a high-fat diet. Get a copy of my second book, *The Fit or Fat Target Diet,* and don't give up!

2. Have you had a body fat test? Do you even know if you're overfat? A lot of big-boned, big-muscled people beat themselves up emotionally and physically by thinking they're too fat when they're actually not fat at all!

3. If, in fact, you really are too fat, you need to exercise more. Twelve minutes of exercise every day is the bare minimum needed to *maintain* present fitness levels. If you're really fat, you need to do a whole lot more.

4. Have you taken your measurements? Have you had a followup body fat test? How do you know you aren't changing? It may be that you're losing fat but at the same time gaining muscle, so your scales register no loss of weight.

5. Have you pulse-monitored your exercise? Are you breathing comfortably? Fat isn't burned when you exercise too hard.

6. Finally, how many years have you been fat? Spend that many years getting unfat. It takes time to change muscle enzymes so that they burn fat well. You've spent many years teaching them how NOT to burn fat. They deserve the same amount of time for reeducation.

Dear Mr. Bailey,
I exercise about one hour a day, running approximately eight miles. I eat a low-fat diet of about 2000 calories a day. I get body fat tested every six months and keep getting the same results: 19 percent. What can I do to lose more fat?
Sue M.
San Diego, California

Dear Sue,
First of all, you need to realize that 19 percent fat is very, very good. Too many people have gotten the wrong idea that they

must have extremely low levels of fat in order to be healthy. But it seems to me your body is saying, "Hey! I like being 19 percent fat and I'm going to resist going lower. If you keep pushing me, I may retaliate by making you get sick all the time. Or I may stop menstruating. Or I may get rid of fat you'd rather keep, like your breast fat." Given the amount of exercise you are doing and your normal calorie intake, you seem to have a "set point" of 19 percent. This is healthy for you. A healthy person doesn't try to change the set point of her calcium levels or hormone levels, does she? I know that sounds like a silly question, but it's just as silly for a person to tamper with his or her fat levels if they are in the range of good health. Your performance and endurance indicate that you are very fit. If your body prefers a 19 percent fat level, so be it.

> Dear Mr. Bailey,
>   I recently had a hysterectomy, and did that ever change my body! I used to be 22 percent fat, and now I can't get it any lower than 28 percent. I'm very diligent about my diet (I keep it at 20–25 percent fat). I've even increased my exercise from thirty minutes to forty-five minutes a day. Help!
>   Rhonda S.
>   Wichita, Kansas

Dear Rhonda,
   You didn't say in your letter, but I suspect you are now taking some kind of hormone replacement drug. A 5 to 10 percent increase in body fat is almost inevitable with these drugs. Female hormones increase body fat. This is why we say healthy women are allowed to be 22 percent fat, while men must shoot for 15 percent. If a man takes female hormones (as protection against a second heart attack, for instance), his body fat increases. Women using birth control pills also have about 2 or 3 percent more fat than when they are not taking them.
   Women who are postmenopausal, either naturally or from a hysterectomy, face another problem if they choose not to use

hormone replacement therapy. The lack of estrogen augments bone loss. They don't gain fat, but they lose lean. This, too, gives a high body fat reading. (The ratio of fat to lean increases, giving a higher percentage of fat even though the actual pounds of fat may be unchanged.)

In any case, since you exercise a lot and watch your diet carefully, please don't try to get back down to 22 percent fat. Accept 28 percent as normal for you, being sure to test yourself occasionally to stay on track.

Dear Mr. Bailey,
   I am sixty-two years old, and I enjoyed your book, but I wish you had written more for us "older folks."
                                    Jim J.
                                    Springfield, Massachusetts

Dear Jim,

Actually, *Fit or Fat* applies to all ages. It doesn't matter whether you're young or old, male or female, white or black. The basic rules and information apply to everyone. People of all ages and races, male and female, need to exercise to control fat, to improve heart and lungs, to ward off depression. Exercise in older people yields additional benefits by slowing the loss of bone minerals and maintaining mobility even as the years pile up.

Do everything that a twenty-year-old does, but do it more slowly. You still need to exercise aerobically. You'll just find that an aerobic pace for you is much slower than it is for a twenty-year-old. Remember that you do not repair as quickly as when you were young. (Even here, however, older people who exercise have an advantage because their repair mechanisms function better than those of people who don't exercise.)

You have all the time in the world now to exercise so why not use it? Take long walks after dinner. While all the kids are in school, use the local pool for a half hour or so of lap swimming. Join a hiking club. The only things you need to do differently from when you were young are to vary your activities more to avoid trauma to any one joint and to allow more recovery time between exercise sessions.

Dear Mr. Bailey,
I was body fat tested and came out 19 percent. How long will it take me to get to 15 percent?
Joseph D.
Los Angeles, California

Dear Joseph,
You didn't provide enough information for me to give you other than a general answer. As a basic rule of thumb, we find that people who exercise aerobically for about thirty to forty-five minutes every other day AND eat a low-fat (20–25 percent fat) diet, around 1800–2000 calories a day for women and 2400–2700 calories a day for men, lose approximately ½ percent body fat per month. In other words, it should take you about eight months to lose 4 percent fat. This is modified by:

1. Your past athletic history. People who have never exercised have more trouble losing fat than "ex-jocks."
2. Your family history of fatness. If fat runs in your family, you'll be much more resistant to fat loss than other people.

Finally, you lose fat more slowly as you get closer and closer to your goal. Very fat people (over 40 percent fat) often drop 1 percent fat a month in the initial stages, but this slows down in time, and the ½ percent a month figure becomes the overall average.

Dear Mr. Bailey,

   My body fat test came out 22 percent fat, which you say is healthy for women. But my thighs still jiggle and have that awful cellulite! I don't believe the test. I'm sure I must be 30 percent.

                                        Brenda A.
                                        Vancouver, British Columbia

Dear Brenda,

   At 22 percent fat, you are carrying somewhere around twenty-five to thirty pounds of fat. Suppose we distributed that fat throughout your body. We'd put three pounds under your skin, about three pounds in your breasts, smear another four pounds around your organs, and slather six pounds throughout your muscles. That leaves about nine to fourteen pounds of fat. Where do women store extra fat? Bingo! Five to seven pounds for each thigh! Healthy men have the same complaint as you, only with them it's their midsection. "How can I be 15 percent fat and still have these love handles?" men say.

   Getting rid of that extra fat is sometimes very difficult. I have seen it disappear in some women when they get their total fat down to 18 or 19 percent. In other women it persists, while the loss of fat from the rest of their body makes them look almost emaciated. If your extra fat is stubborn, you might consider liposuction. Plastic surgeons groan when very obese people want all their fat sucked away. But a fit, lean woman or man with a specific irreversible fat deposit is ideal for such surgery.

   Do keep in mind that liposuction does nothing to correct "cellulite," that puckered-skin condition seen in some women. Fair-skinned women seem to have this skin type more than darker-skinned women. Removing the fat under cellulite-type skin will reduce the size of your thigh but will not usually change the puckering. Sometimes building up the muscle underneath the skin will help smooth it out.

33

Why Not Now?

I won't tell you that getting used to daily exercise is a bed of roses. There are times when the best of us would rather quit, put up our feet, and dream of a diet or a pill that will make us healthy. But health doesn't come in a bottle or a diet.

Even the best diet combined with the most potent vitamins will never tune up your muscles the way good exercise will. It seems a shame to put expensive fuel in a poor machine. If your car isn't running well, do you drive all around town looking for better and better gasoline, or do you have your car tuned up? Remember, it's your muscles that burn most of the calories you eat. It's largely your muscle chemistry that determines whether that good diet or those vitamins get properly used or just wasted.

It would be nice if everyone had the opportunity to get weighed under water occasionally to determine just how fat he or she is. Lacking this information, you can't always tell whether you are overfat or not. Occasionally we see people in our clinic who look overfat but who are just big-boned and big-muscled without much fat at all.

The point is, it is impossible for me to tell you in a book what weight to shoot for, but it is equally impossible for you or your doctor or a table to tell you what weight to shoot for. If you have been reading this book thoughtfully, you should be convinced by now that the cause of excess fat is poor muscle tone. You should stop thinking about weight and start thinking about muscle. You should think about your level of physical fitness and measure changes in that.

Don't ask how much you should weigh. Stop shooting for an ideal weight! Shoot for health, for being physically fit. When you exercise, don't think about how many calories you are burning; think about your enzymes. When I do my morning run, I mutter under my breath, "Grow, you enzymes, grow!" If you can, check your blood pressure once in a while to see if it comes down as you get healthier. By all means check your resting pulse. The easiest thing of all to check is your measurements. In both men and women, the waist decreases as the abdominal muscles flatten out. Hip and thigh measurements in women decrease quickly with exercise.

These simple measurements may seem unsophisticated, but they are far better measures of health than your weight. If you want more encouragement, ask your doctor to check other health factors from time to time. For instance, if you tend to have a trace of sugar in your urine, it will decrease with good exercise. Hypoglycemia decreases with exercise, as does high blood triglyceride. Don't be impatient; these improvements take time — at least a year, sometimes four or five years in older people.

Having tuned-up muscles doesn't mean that you have to become an athlete. It means you'll have more energy and more drive, and your body will use food more efficiently and convert less of it to fat.

One reason for the high dropout rate from exercise and weight loss programs is that people have been told too often that it's easy. Losing weight and becoming fit is NOT easy. I cringe when weight control programs advertise how easy it is to lose weight. However, something that is hard is not necessarily unpleasant. Ask any outdoorsman how he feels after an all-day hike in the mountains. Was it hard? Definitely! Was it unpleasant? No!

Accomplishments that take effort give us tremendous satisfaction. Parenting is hard, but it's not unpleasant. Building your own home is an extremely difficult — but extremely satisfying — task. If you're about to start an exercise and fat control program, don't fool yourself into thinking it will be easy. Approach it in the same way you would approach being a parent, going to college, or hiking up a mountain. It's going to be tough, but it will be worth it.

So start exercising! Like the rest of us, you will falter from time to time, but persist, and gradually your whole physical and mental well-being will improve. Be sure to pulse-monitor and "talk-test" your efforts so that you won't overdo, so that you can avoid much of the muscle pain that used to be a regular part of unguided exercise. Reversing twenty years of fatty muscle degeneration may take months, even years in some cases, but hang in there; lots of us are with you. I mean, *really* with you.

Join those of us who are proud to be getting the most out of the bodies we were given. Start now!

The New Aerobics Logbook

A Realistic Approach to Exercise

The New Aerobics Logbook is for everybody —
young, old, male, female. It is designed to help you
achieve maximum physical fitness with a minimum
of stress. The emphasis is on TIME, not distance.

Most exercise programs measure distance versus time: how far can you run, cycle, row, or whatever in a certain amount of time? The major flaw in such programs is that in order to earn more miles, people often exercise too hard and too fast. They exceed their comfortable aerobic pace in order to squeeze in that extra quarter-mile.

Studies have shown that for the greatest cardiovascular improvement and most efficient fat burning, exercise should fall in the range at which the heart beats between 65 percent and 80 percent of its maximum. The exercise should be at a rate that causes deep breathing, not gasping, and allows you to talk in halting phrases. This is AEROBIC exercise; improvement comes from increasing the time you spend doing it, not from increasing the speed.

You will notice that in my logbook there's no place to keep track of distance. You measure only the time you spend exercising. You earn *minutes,* not miles.

HOW TO USE <u>THE NEW AEROBICS LOGBOOK</u>

Each Week Record Your Minutes of Exercise

In my original Aerobics Logbook you earned minutes only when you exercised aerobically. This confused a lot of people. "Doesn't tennis count for anything?" they asked. Or "Does that mean I can count only the first part of my aerobics class, when I'm on my feet, and the last part, when I'm doing floor work, doesn't count?" We now know that ANY type of activity is good for you. The racket sports yield lots of aerobic benefits. Weight lifting and body building, although they are not aerobic, add fat-burning muscle. Even playing Frisbee or softball with your friends on weekends is good for you.

In my New Aerobics Logbook you earn minutes for *any* exercise activity. Each week you aim for a certain number of exercise minutes, of which a minimum amount must be AEROBIC MINUTES. To this you can add NONAEROBIC MINUTES of exercise such as tennis (which is too stop-and-go to be considered aerobic), or weight lifting (which is too intense to be considered aerobic), or golf (which is too slow to be considered aerobic). All of these nonaerobic activities are good for you, but in producing cardiovascular improvement and fat-burning improvement they are *not as efficient* as aerobic activity.

Each Month Record Your Measurements

Although I know you won't be able to resist weighing yourself, I have not provided a place to record your weight. Changes in weight are somewhat meaningless since you don't know whether you're losing (or gaining) fat or muscle. Of much greater significance are changes in body measurements. Typically, men store fat around their middles and women store fat in their thighs and hips. At the end of each month, measure your fat storage areas to see if they are getting smaller.

Every Three Months Take My Aerobic Fitness Test

This test is described on page 164. Let me stress again — THIS IS NOT A TEST TO SEE HOW FAST YOU CAN RUN!!! It MUST be done at a comfortable aerobic pace to be of any value. If you're just starting an exercise program, I recommend that you test yourself every month. After that, do it about every three months. You should find that it takes you less time to comfortably cover a mile each month. At first the decreases will be noticeable — ten, twenty, even thirty seconds less. Later on, there'll be only small improvements or perhaps no change at all. That's okay. If you've reached one of these plateaus, you can sometimes add more minutes to your weekly routine or add wind sprints once or twice a week to get an improvement in the fitness test. But remember this caution! If your fitness test comes out *worse*, ease up on your exercise program! This is your body's way of letting you know you're exercising too hard.

Every Six to Twelve Months Measure Your Body Fat

Try to find a place in your town where you can have a body fat test, perhaps at the YMCA, a college physical education department, or a gym or health club. You should keep track of three numbers: your body fat percentage, your pounds of lean, and your pounds of fat. You should then recheck yourself every six to twelve months. Is your fat going up or down? What's happening to your lean? If you were ill for a prolonged time, did it affect your lean? Did that Caribbean cruise last winter play havoc with your fat? How is your new exercise program affecting your body composition?

The Body Machine's Care Schedule

	MONTH											
	1	2	3	4	5	6	7	8	9	10	11	12
Minimum minutes of AEROBIC exercise	240	240	240	240	240	240	240	240	240	240	240	240
Total minimum minutes of exercise (aerobic and nonaerobic)	360	360	360	360	360	360	360	360	360	360	360	360
Check body measurements	•	•	•	•	•	•	•	•	•	•	•	•
Do aerobic fitness test	•			•			•			•		
Measure body fat	•						•					

A word about diet: I've written two books about low-fat, high-fiber eating; I refer my readers to *The Fit-or-Fat Target Diet* and *Fit-or-Fat Target Recipes* for more detailed information. In general, you should try to eat a diet that is approximately 25 percent fat. If you need to lose five to fifteen pounds of fat, decrease the total fat in your diet to 20 percent. If you are very fat, decrease it to 10 to 15 percent fat.

THE AEROBIC FITNESS TEST

Before you take this test, you must first determine *your* correct exercise heart rate. Too many people accept a target heart rate for themselves from some average in a chart or book or from an exercise instructor. But those averages don't consider that *your* heart might beat faster or slower than normal or that you might be on a medication that affects your heart rate.

If I were helping you find your correct aerobic pace, I would do the following. I would have you walk on a treadmill with a heart rate monitor strapped around your chest. Then I would gradually increase the speed of the treadmill while I carefully noted your breathing. When you reached the point where you were breathing deeply — but not panting — and were still able to talk to me, haltingly, not fluently, I would record the pulse rate indicated on the monitor as your "target" aerobic heart rate. At this point an elite marathoner might be running an "aerobic" five-minute mile while a fat, sedentary person might be barely walking a twenty-minute mile.

Since I can't do this test for you, *you* must determine your own target rate by *first* establishing a comfortable exercise pace that you can maintain steadily and then taking your pulse during that comfortable pace. Please be practical! Don't concern yourself with how fast your friends run or what the books tell you to do. Just find out what's comfortable *for you*. For 60 percent of you, your comfortable exercise heart rate will fall in the training range described in Chapters 11 and 12, which is 65–80 percent of your maximum heart rate:

$$(220 - \text{age}) \times .65 \text{ and } .80 = \text{training zone}$$

About 40 percent of you who do this test will be surprised to find that your aerobic heart rate determined by this method is quite different from that shown in charts or derived from the formula. Don't worry about this. If you are breathing deeply but not panting, if you can carry on limited conversation, and *if you are comfortable,* then this is your correct pace.

Repeat this routine for three or four days until you can consistently hold your pulse in your training zone. Some of you jocks may find this pace a little slow. Never mind. You should be able to stop at any time in the middle of your exercise, take a six-second pulse, multiply by ten, and consistently get within four beats of your aerobic pulse.

Now! TO DO THE TEST:

Find a flat, level mile. Maybe use a high school track, which is usually a quarter-mile around, or measure one mile on a road with your car. Warm up by walking rapidly or jogging slowly for five to eight minutes, then start your aerobic pace and time yourself as you cover the mile WITHOUT going faster than the aerobic pace (or heart rate) you have been practicing.

This test produces just one all-important number! *How many minutes does it take you to cover one mile without exceeding your training heart rate?* _____ minutes

NOTE! Accidents can happen during exercise. That's a fact. The vast majority of people, if they perform this test properly, at a *comfortable* aerobic level, will experience no difficulty. Nonetheless, something *could* happen, and you have to decide for yourself if you want to take the risk. Remember what I said about a comfortable exercise level: if it stops being comfortable, pay attention and slow down or stop. I feel that your personal risk if you *don't* undertake an exercise program is far greater than if you *do*. BUT! I don't want to be liable for your having a problem with exercise.

I expect that you will want to repeat this test every three months to measure your progress. Each time your heart rate should be the same and your breathing level the same. But the time to cover a mile should go down (or up) as your fitness level goes up (or down).

KEEPING TRACK OF YOUR WEEKLY MINUTES

Regular maintenance: At least 60 AEROBIC minutes per week, spread out over at least three days. Plus at least 30 more minutes, either aerobic or nonaerobic.

Minimum maintenance (for the times you're too busy to do more): At least 60 AEROBIC minutes per week, spread out over at least three days.

Need to lose 5–15 pounds of fat: At least 70 AEROBIC minutes per week, spread out over at least three days. Plus at least 60 more minutes, aerobic and/or nonaerobic.

Need to lose more than 15 pounds of fat: At least *two* 12-minute AEROBIC sessions a day, five days a week. Plus at least 20 minutes per day, aerobic and/or nonaerobic, on the other two days.

Need to gain muscle: 30 minutes of AEROBIC exercise three days a week. Work up to 45–60 minutes of weight lifting/body building three days a week (but not on the same day as the aerobic exercise).

Fifty-plus years old: 30 minutes of AEROBIC exercise every other day; switch exercises every other day.

Cardiac impairment: 30 minutes of AEROBIC exercise every other day, with heart rate not above 75 percent of maximum. *Caution! Consult your physician before starting an exercise program.*

AEROBIC EXERCISES

WALKING · JOGGING · RUNNING · BICYCLING · ROWING · CROSS-COUNTRY SKIING · SWIMMING · AEROBIC DANCING · STAIR CLIMBING · JUMPING ROPE · BENCH STEPPING · MINI-TRAMPOLINE · ROLLER SKATING · TREADMILL · HIKING

or anything you do that:
- is steady and nonstop
- is in your training range
- lasts a minimum of 12 minutes
- uses the big muscles in the lower body

NONAEROBIC EXERCISES

TENNIS · RACQUETBALL · HANDBALL · SOFTBALL · GOLF · DANCING · DOWNHILL SKIING · BASKETBALL · WEIGHT LIFTING · BODY BUILDING · FLOOR EXERCISES · HORSEBACK RIDING · FRISBEE

or anything you do that is active but is too stop-and-go or too fast or too slow to be aerobic.

Maintenance Record

Month	Minutes of aerobic exercise (every month)	Minutes of total exercise (every month)	Body measurements (every month)	Aerobic fitness test (every 3 mos.)	Body fat (every 6 mos.)
1	Week 1 ____ Week 2 ____ Week 3 ____ Week 4 ____ Total ____	Week 1 ____ Week 2 ____ Week 3 ____ Week 4 ____ Total ____	Men: waist ____ Women: hips ____ right thigh ____	1 mile in _____ minutes	% fat ____ lbs. fat ____ lbs. lean ____
2	Week 1 ____ Week 2 ____ Week 3 ____ Week 4 ____ Total ____	Week 1 ____ Week 2 ____ Week 3 ____ Week 4 ____ Total ____	Men: waist ____ Women: hips ____ right thigh ____		
3	Week 1 ____ Week 2 ____ Week 3 ____ Week 4 ____ Total ____	Week 1 ____ Week 2 ____ Week 3 ____ Week 4 ____ Total ____	Men: waist ____ Women: hips ____ right thigh ____		
4	Week 1 ____ Week 2 ____ Week 3 ____ Week 4 ____ Total ____	Week 1 ____ Week 2 ____ Week 3 ____ Week 4 ____ Total ____	Men: waist ____ Women: hips ____ right thigh ____	1 mile in _____ minutes	
5	Week 1 ____ Week 2 ____ Week 3 ____ Week 4 ____ Total ____	Week 1 ____ Week 2 ____ Week 3 ____ Week 4 ____ Total ____	Men: waist ____ Women: hips ____ right thigh ____		
6	Week 1 ____ Week 2 ____ Week 3 ____ Week 4 ____ Total ____	Week 1 ____ Week 2 ____ Week 3 ____ Week 4 ____ Total ____	Men: waist ____ Women: hips ____ right thigh ____		

Maintenance Record

Month	Minutes of aerobic exercise (every month)	Minutes of total exercise (every month)	Body measurements (every month)	Aerobic fitness test (every 3 mos.)	Body fat (every 6 mos.)
1	Week 1 ____ Week 2 ____ Week 3 ____ Week 4 ____ Total ____	Week 1 ____ Week 2 ____ Week 3 ____ Week 4 ____ Total ____	Men: waist ____ Women: hips ____ right thigh ____	1 mile in _____ minutes	% fat ____ lbs. fat ____ lbs. lean ____
2	Week 1 ____ Week 2 ____ Week 3 ____ Week 4 ____ Total ____	Week 1 ____ Week 2 ____ Week 3 ____ Week 4 ____ Total ____	Men: waist ____ Women: hips ____ right thigh ____		
3	Week 1 ____ Week 2 ____ Week 3 ____ Week 4 ____ Total ____	Week 1 ____ Week 2 ____ Week 3 ____ Week 4 ____ Total ____	Men: waist ____ Women: hips ____ right thigh ____		
4	Week 1 ____ Week 2 ____ Week 3 ____ Week 4 ____ Total ____	Week 1 ____ Week 2 ____ Week 3 ____ Week 4 ____ Total ____	Men: waist ____ Women: hips ____ right thigh ____	1 mile in _____ minutes	
5	Week 1 ____ Week 2 ____ Week 3 ____ Week 4 ____ Total ____	Week 1 ____ Week 2 ____ Week 3 ____ Week 4 ____ Total ____	Men: waist ____ Women: hips ____ right thigh ____		
6	Week 1 ____ Week 2 ____ Week 3 ____ Week 4 ____ Total ____	Week 1 ____ Week 2 ____ Week 3 ____ Week 4 ____ Total ____	Men: waist ____ Women: hips ____ right thigh ____		

Maintenance Record

Month	Minutes of aerobic exercise (every month)	Minutes of total exercise (every month)	Body measurements (every month)	Aerobic fitness test (every 3 mos.)	Body fat (every 6 mos.)
1	Week 1 ____ Week 2 ____ Week 3 ____ Week 4 ____ Total ____	Week 1 ____ Week 2 ____ Week 3 ____ Week 4 ____ Total ____	Men: waist ____ Women: hips ____ right thigh ____	1 mile in _____ minutes	% fat ____ lbs. fat ____ lbs. lean ____
2	Week 1 ____ Week 2 ____ Week 3 ____ Week 4 ____ Total ____	Week 1 ____ Week 2 ____ Week 3 ____ Week 4 ____ Total ____	Men: waist ____ Women: hips ____ right thigh ____		
3	Week 1 ____ Week 2 ____ Week 3 ____ Week 4 ____ Total ____	Week 1 ____ Week 2 ____ Week 3 ____ Week 4 ____ Total ____	Men: waist ____ Women: hips ____ right thigh ____		
4	Week 1 ____ Week 2 ____ Week 3 ____ Week 4 ____ Total ____	Week 1 ____ Week 2 ____ Week 3 ____ Week 4 ____ Total ____	Men: waist ____ Women: hips ____ right thigh ____	1 mile in _____ minutes	
5	Week 1 ____ Week 2 ____ Week 3 ____ Week 4 ____ Total ____	Week 1 ____ Week 2 ____ Week 3 ____ Week 4 ____ Total ____	Men: waist ____ Women: hips ____ right thigh ____		
6	Week 1 ____ Week 2 ____ Week 3 ____ Week 4 ____ Total ____	Week 1 ____ Week 2 ____ Week 3 ____ Week 4 ____ Total ____	Men: waist ____ Women: hips ____ right thigh ____		

Maintenance Record

Month	Minutes of aerobic exercise (every month)	Minutes of total exercise (every month)	Body measurements (every month)	Aerobic fitness test (every 3 mos.)	Body fat (every 6 mos.)
1	Week 1 ____ Week 2 ____ Week 3 ____ Week 4 ____ Total ____	Week 1 ____ Week 2 ____ Week 3 ____ Week 4 ____ Total ____	Men: waist ____ Women: hips ____ right thigh ____	1 mile in _____ minutes	% fat ____ lbs. fat ____ lbs. lean ____
2	Week 1 ____ Week 2 ____ Week 3 ____ Week 4 ____ Total ____	Week 1 ____ Week 2 ____ Week 3 ____ Week 4 ____ Total ____	Men: waist ____ Women: hips ____ right thigh ____		
3	Week 1 ____ Week 2 ____ Week 3 ____ Week 4 ____ Total ____	Week 1 ____ Week 2 ____ Week 3 ____ Week 4 ____ Total ____	Men: waist ____ Women: hips ____ right thigh ____		
4	Week 1 ____ Week 2 ____ Week 3 ____ Week 4 ____ Total ____	Week 1 ____ Week 2 ____ Week 3 ____ Week 4 ____ Total ____	Men: waist ____ Women: hips ____ right thigh ____	1 mile in _____ minutes	
5	Week 1 ____ Week 2 ____ Week 3 ____ Week 4 ____ Total ____	Week 1 ____ Week 2 ____ Week 3 ____ Week 4 ____ Total ____	Men: waist ____ Women: hips ____ right thigh ____		
6	Week 1 ____ Week 2 ____ Week 3 ____ Week 4 ____ Total ____	Week 1 ____ Week 2 ____ Week 3 ____ Week 4 ____ Total ____	Men: waist ____ Women: hips ____ right thigh ____		

Maintenance Record

Month	Minutes of aerobic exercise (every month)	Minutes of total exercise (every month)	Body measurements (every month)	Aerobic fitness test (every 3 mos.)	Body fat (every 6 mos.)
1	Week 1 ____ Week 2 ____ Week 3 ____ Week 4 ____ Total ____	Week 1 ____ Week 2 ____ Week 3 ____ Week 4 ____ Total ____	Men: waist ____ Women: hips ____ right thigh ____	1 mile in _____ minutes	% fat ____ lbs. fat ____ lbs. lean ____
2	Week 1 ____ Week 2 ____ Week 3 ____ Week 4 ____ Total ____	Week 1 ____ Week 2 ____ Week 3 ____ Week 4 ____ Total ____	Men: waist ____ Women: hips ____ right thigh ____		
3	Week 1 ____ Week 2 ____ Week 3 ____ Week 4 ____ Total ____	Week 1 ____ Week 2 ____ Week 3 ____ Week 4 ____ Total ____	Men: waist ____ Women: hips ____ right thigh ____		
4	Week 1 ____ Week 2 ____ Week 3 ____ Week 4 ____ Total ____	Week 1 ____ Week 2 ____ Week 3 ____ Week 4 ____ Total ____	Men: waist ____ Women: hips ____ right thigh ____	1 mile in _____ minutes	
5	Week 1 ____ Week 2 ____ Week 3 ____ Week 4 ____ Total ____	Week 1 ____ Week 2 ____ Week 3 ____ Week 4 ____ Total ____	Men: waist ____ Women: hips ____ right thigh ____		
6	Week 1 ____ Week 2 ____ Week 3 ____ Week 4 ____ Total ____	Week 1 ____ Week 2 ____ Week 3 ____ Week 4 ____ Total ____	Men: waist ____ Women: hips ____ right thigh ____		

Maintenance Record

Month	Minutes of aerobic exercise (every month)	Minutes of total exercise (every month)	Body measurements (every month)	Aerobic fitness test (every 3 mos.)	Body fat (every 6 mos.)
1	Week 1 ____ Week 2 ____ Week 3 ____ Week 4 ____ Total ____	Week 1 ____ Week 2 ____ Week 3 ____ Week 4 ____ Total ____	Men: waist ____ Women: hips ____ right thigh ____	1 mile in _____ minutes	% fat ____ lbs. fat ____ lbs. lean ____
2	Week 1 ____ Week 2 ____ Week 3 ____ Week 4 ____ Total ____	Week 1 ____ Week 2 ____ Week 3 ____ Week 4 ____ Total ____	Men: waist ____ Women: hips ____ right thigh ____		
3	Week 1 ____ Week 2 ____ Week 3 ____ Week 4 ____ Total ____	Week 1 ____ Week 2 ____ Week 3 ____ Week 4 ____ Total ____	Men: waist ____ Women: hips ____ right thigh ____		
4	Week 1 ____ Week 2 ____ Week 3 ____ Week 4 ____ Total ____	Week 1 ____ Week 2 ____ Week 3 ____ Week 4 ____ Total ____	Men: waist ____ Women: hips ____ right thigh ____	1 mile in _____ minutes	
5	Week 1 ____ Week 2 ____ Week 3 ____ Week 4 ____ Total ____	Week 1 ____ Week 2 ____ Week 3 ____ Week 4 ____ Total ____	Men: waist ____ Women: hips ____ right thigh ____		
6	Week 1 ____ Week 2 ____ Week 3 ____ Week 4 ____ Total ____	Week 1 ____ Week 2 ____ Week 3 ____ Week 4 ____ Total ____	Men: waist ____ Women: hips ____ right thigh ____		

Weekly Record of Exercise Minutes*

Date	Type of exercise	Aerobic?	Minutes	Nonaerobic?	Minutes

Total for week:

AEROBIC minutes: _____**

Nonaerobic minutes: _____

Total minutes: _____

(Transfer these numbers to your maintenance record)

*Please make several copies of this record so you'll have enough for many weeks.
**Remember, aerobic minutes include *only* the time when you are actually exercising in your training range and you are breathing deeply but not panting. Don't include warm-up or cool-down minutes or time spent doing wind sprints. (However, you *can* include these as *nonaerobic* minutes of exercise.)

Weekly Record of Exercise Minutes*

Date	Type of exercise	Aerobic?	Minutes	Nonaerobic?	Minutes

Total for week:

AEROBIC minutes: _____ **

Nonaerobic minutes: _____

Total minutes: _____

(Transfer these numbers to your maintenance record)

*Please make several copies of this record so you'll have enough for many weeks.
**Remember, aerobic minutes include *only* the time when you are actually exercising in your training range and you are breathing deeply but not panting. Don't include warm-up or cool-down minutes or time spent doing wind sprints. (However, you *can* include these as *nonaerobic* minutes of exercise.)

Weekly Record of Exercise Minutes*

Date	Type of exercise	Aerobic?	Minutes	Nonaerobic?	Minutes

Total for week:

AEROBIC minutes: _____**

Nonaerobic minutes: _____

Total minutes: _____

(Transfer these numbers to your maintenance record)

*Please make several copies of this record so you'll have enough for many weeks.
**Remember, aerobic minutes include *only* the time when you are actually exercising in your training range and you are breathing deeply but not panting. Don't include warm-up or cool-down minutes or time spent doing wind sprints. (However, you *can* include these as *nonaerobic* minutes of exercise.)

Weekly Record of Exercise Minutes*

Date	Type of exercise	Aerobic?	Minutes	Nonaerobic?	Minutes

Total for week:

AEROBIC minutes: _____**

Nonaerobic minutes: _____

Total minutes: _____

(Transfer these numbers to your maintenance record)

*Please make several copies of this record so you'll have enough for many weeks.
**Remember, aerobic minutes include *only* the time when you are actually exercising in your training range and you are breathing deeply but not panting. Don't include warm-up or cool-down minutes or time spent doing wind sprints. (However, you *can* include these as *nonaerobic* minutes of exercise.)

Weekly Record of Exercise Minutes*

Date	Type of exercise	Aerobic?	Minutes	Nonaerobic?	Minutes

Total for week:

AEROBIC **minutes:** _____ **

Nonaerobic minutes: _____

Total minutes: _____

(Transfer these numbers to your maintenance record)

*Please make several copies of this record so you'll have enough for many weeks.

**Remember, aerobic minutes include *only* the time when you are actually exercising in your training range and you are breathing deeply but not panting. Don't include warm-up or cool-down minutes or time spent doing wind sprints. (However, you *can* include these as *nonaerobic* minutes of exercise.)

Weekly Record of Exercise Minutes*

Date	Type of exercise	Aerobic?	Minutes	Nonaerobic?	Minutes

Total for week:

AEROBIC minutes: _____**

Nonaerobic minutes: _____

Total minutes: _____

(Transfer these numbers to your maintenance record)

*Please make several copies of this record so you'll have enough for many weeks.
**Remember, aerobic minutes include *only* the time when you are actually exercising in your training range and you are breathing deeply but not panting. Don't include warm-up or cool-down minutes or time spent doing wind sprints. (However, you *can* include these as *nonaerobic* minutes of exercise.)